Praise for
Love Food and Live Well

"In *Love Food and Live Well*, Chantel Hobbs helps readers re-create their lives from the inside out. As you turn the pages of this book, you can't help but feel that Chantel is right there with you to guide and inspire every step in your quest to eat better, move more, and enjoy a more fulfilled and more healthful life."

—ELISA ZIED, MS, RD, CDN, regular contributor to msnbc.com
and GALTime.com; author of *Nutrition at Your Fingertips*
and *Feed Your Family Right!*

"Behind Chantel's extraordinary story and unquestioned expertise is a heart that sets her apart. Regardless of whom she encounters, she lives for the opportunity to help them discover their fullest and fittest potential. As you read *Love Food and Live Well*, it will become clear that Chantel is doing what God created her to do. How refreshing to find a fitness expert who is devoted to changing lives on the inside as well as the outside!"

—BOB COY, pastor of Calvary Chapel, Fort Lauderdale

"Chantel Hobbs uses wit, wisdom, and poignant insights to open our eyes regarding our health and well-being. With helpful tips, exercises, recipes, and workout plans, Chantel has put together a perfect plan that anyone can follow. And she points out that allowing God to take control is the only way to live a life that will make everything else fall into place."

—MIKE HUCKABEE, former Arkansas governor; author of *Quit
Digging Your Grave with a Knife and Fork;* host of *Huckabee*

"*Love Food and Live Well* inspires you to focus on what's good, what's true, and what works. If you have ever felt trapped and miserable, Chantel Hobbs will show you how to surrender your life and gain control of what matters most. Filled with real-life success stories, *Love Food and Live Well* will help you begin the journey that will change your life forever."

—MILES METTLER, PhD in exercise and wellness; general manager of Saint Mary's Center for Health and Fitness, Reno, Nevada

Chantel Hobbs

author of *Never Say Diet*

Lose Weight, Get Fit, & Taste Life
at Its Very Best

Love
Food
&
Live Well

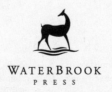

WATERBROOK
PRESS

Love Food and Live Well
Published by WaterBrook Press
12265 Oracle Boulevard, Suite 200
Colorado Springs, Colorado 80921

This book is not intended as a substitute for the advice and care of your physician, and as with any other fitness, diet, or nutrition plan, you should use proper discretion, in consultation with your physician, in utilizing the information presented. The author and the publisher expressly disclaim responsibility for any adverse effects that may result from the use or application of the information contained in this book.

All Scripture quotations, unless otherwise indicated, are taken from the New King James Version®. Copyright © 1982 by Thomas Nelson Inc. Used by permission. All rights reserved. Scripture quotations marked (MSG) are taken from The Message by Eugene H. Peterson. Copyright © 1993, 1994, 1995, 1996, 2000, 2001, 2002. Used by permission of NavPress Publishing Group. All rights reserved. Scripture quotations marked (NIV) are taken from the Holy Bible, New International Version®. NIV®. Copyright © 1973, 1978, 1984 by Biblica Inc.™ Used by permission of Zondervan. All rights reserved worldwide. www.zondervan.com.

Details in some anecdotes and stories have been changed to protect the identities of the persons involved.

ISBN 978-0-307-45785-1
ISBN 978-0-307-45786-8 (electronic)

Copyright © 2010 by Chantel Hobbs
Appendix copyright © 2011 by Chantel Hobbs
Interior exercise photographs © 2010 by Helene Kopel
Photo on page 157 © 2010 by Ashley Hobbs
Photo on page 145 © 2010 by Marcos M. Sendon

All rights reserved. No part of this book may be reproduced or transmitted in any form or by any means, electronic or mechanical, including photocopying and recording, or by any information storage and retrieval system, without permission in writing from the publisher.

Published in the United States by WaterBrook Multnomah, an imprint of the Crown Publishing Group, a division of Random House Inc., New York.

WATERBROOK and its deer colophon are registered trademarks of Random House Inc.

The Library of Congress cataloged the hardcover edition as follows:
Hobbs, Chantel.
   Love food and live well : lose weight, get fit, and taste life at its very best / Chantel Hobbs.
      p. cm.
   Includes bibliographical references.
   ISBN 978-0-307-45784-4 — ISBN 978-0-307-45786-8 (electronic)
   1. Weight loss. 2. Physical fitness. 3. Food habits. I. Title.
   RM222.2.H5728 2010
   613.7—dc22
                          2010027091

Printed in the United States of America
2011—First Trade Paperback Edition

10 9 8 7 6 5 4 3 2 1

SPECIAL SALES
Most WaterBrook Multnomah books are available at special quantity discounts when purchased in bulk by corporations, organizations, and special-interest groups. Custom imprinting or excerpting can also be done to fit special needs. For information, please e-mail SpecialMarkets@WaterBrookMultnomah.com or call 1-800-603-7051.

For the lost

———

Some of us know what it feels like to be alone in a crowded room.
This book is for you. May you find the love you long for
and the acceptance you've needed your entire life.
Believe me: neither a scale nor a pair of jeans nor a human being
can provide it.
I pray that after reading this book, you will find the answer.
It is the ultimate deal of a lifetime,
and it can be yours today!

CONTENTS

Contents

FOREWORD

You need to meet Chantel Hobbs.

I'll do my best, but it won't be the typical, surface-level introduction. Chantel is a mom, yes; and a loving wife, yes; and she now makes her living as a writer. All those things are wonderful, but not why you should meet her.

You should meet her because she's *been there*. And by "there" I mean "here," for many of us. "Here" is a place where we're utterly heartbroken. We're not who we want to be, frustrated with how we look and feel, maybe even disgusted. To know Chantel, you will know her story and how God took not only two hundred excess pounds from her body, but He took away much more in guilt and disappointment with herself.

So, like I say, she's been there. And she's seen what can happen—what works in our relationship with food and what doesn't. And she's experienced how God sees us, which is so much more clearly than we see ourselves.

She's an expert, yes, but she's not just an expert. In Chantel, you have much better.

You have a friend.

Experts can be wonderful, of course. So wonderful, in fact, that they inspire you…to just give up. They're too awesome, too amazing, too "together," and too unapproachable. You spend time with them, and you're left impressed—but only with them. You're left depressed about yourself.

As you'll find in this book, Chantel is just the opposite. When she joins me on my radio show, we are flooded with callers. And to each one, she's unfailingly patient and compassionate. She listens and she nods, because she's been where they now are. She knows why they're calling, and that's not for mere advice: they're looking for hope.

Make friends with Chantel, and she will point you to Hope.

—Brant Hansen, host of the syndicated radio show *Mornings with Brant,* www.morningswithbrant.com

ACKNOWLEDGMENTS

Friends, this book was written out of my own desperate need for the deal of a lifetime!

To my husband, Keith: Babe, thank you for giving me the space for God to do what only He can do. I adore watching you "be daddy" to our children. The way you love me could never be compared…

To my daughter Ashley: As you venture into young adulthood, I feel blessed to call you "my teenager." Your heart for the least of these is a beautiful thing to witness. We can't wait to watch God continue to reveal His unique will for your life.

To my daughter Kayla: I see so much of me in you. Not only does it make me smile; it makes me feel quite humble. I know God will use your thoughtfulness and willingness to serve in mighty ways. Always be proud of who He created you to be.

To my son Jake: You are so very special to me. Not to mention insanely funny and witty! Your take on most situations offers the entire family a great opportunity to laugh together. I love cooking with you and seeing you catch all those big bass!

To my son Luke: You are my "son-shine"! Even though your entrance was a surprise to us, God handpicked you for our home. Everyone isn't always being mean to you, by the way. They are just jealous because you're the baby!

To my mother: You're a brave and beautiful woman. I am constantly in awe of your ability to let life happen and still trust God. Thank you for displaying true faith and utter dependence on your Savior.

To my dad: You are a three-ring circus on a stage and disguised as Johnny Cash or Elvis most of the time. Thanks for teaching me how to laugh more and love life. You're also a wonderful husband and father.

To my in-laws, Ken and Linda: You truly run the race well. While sanctification may require a lifetime, your lives make me want to keep my foot on the gas! Your son is a remarkable man. Thank you for sacrificing and investing in his life as you have. Our children and I now reap what you have sown. My gratitude cannot be expressed in words.

To my dear friend Kerri: Your arrival back in my life, in a fancy bathroom on a late night in Manhattan, was more than a miracle. It was a kiss from God. Thank you for always letting me "bring it" and mostly for keeping it real—even if it meant helping me face my funk. There's no one I'd rather face it with than you.

To Ron Lee: You are a wonderful editor. I appreciate your ear and willingness to let me ramble. I value your gift more than you know.

Thank you to the entire staff at WaterBrook Press: From sales to marketing and publicity, you all have a passion for books that can make a difference. Thank you for your encouragement in all I do.

To my agent, Chip MacGregor: Thanks for being a friend and for supporting my mission of faith, food, and fitness.

To Christy, David, Michael, Kenny, Kevin, and Kris: I am in awe of God's providence in our lives. We are so blessed! I pray you will each seek His will and freely abandon your own will on a regular basis. It has been amazing to watch us all grow up and have families of our own. Let's stay the course and keep Christ the center of our homes.

Thank you to the many people I have met in the past few years who have been so gracious. I am honored that you trust me enough to share your struggles and pain. You are always in my heart and on my mind. You are the reason I seek God while I write. Please pray as you begin to read this book, and allow Him to set you free. He's whispering your name...

To my Rescuer: Thank You, thank You for giving me mercy. I have done nothing to deserve it. I pray I will never hesitate to show compassion and understanding to those who come across my path. Please help me love my neighbor better all the time. Amazing grace is more than a sweet sound. Thank You for saving a wretch like me.

Love Food as Never Before

Most days I don't go looking for adventure, but somehow one finds me. My life is a great adventure, and today is no exception. I had intended to write the introduction to this book weeks ago, but it didn't happen. Then my flight from New York to Fort Lauderdale was canceled, so suddenly I have time on my hands.

After spending the night in a hotel, I'm sitting on a bench in Lower Manhattan, and it's barely daylight. I'm one block from Wall Street, cabs are speeding by, and the people who pull the levers of high finance keep streaming out of a nearby subway station. It's crazy how appropriate all this is, because in this book you and I are going to talk about deals.

We'll look at the deal the world has been selling us all our lives—the message that we're not good enough, not pretty enough, not thin enough, and just basically that we're not enough. Then we'll talk about your particular deal. (Many of you have already told me your stories, so I have a good idea of what you've been struggling with.) And after that, I'll tell you about my past deal involving a pair of jeans, living in constant fear of embarrassment, and much more. Thankfully, that's all behind me.

Then I want to introduce you to the deal of a lifetime, which is available at no cost to you—at least no financial cost—and which has the power to change your life if you choose to go there.

You've heard all the hype, I know. You've been lied to by the diet industry. You've wasted your hard-earned money on gadgets and miracle pills and supplements that were supposed to melt the fat away. Right? So you're understandably skeptical about me or anyone else who promises you a deal that will deliver what the other programs failed to do.

I was skeptical too, until I developed the program that made it possible for me to lose 200 pounds, tone my muscles, and maintain a healthy weight while pursuing a fun and active life. I described this program in my first book, *Never Say Diet*. Now every day I hear from people who have adopted it and lost 15, 50, or 150 pounds. Their lives will never be the same.

I expanded on that program and put it within easy reach for anyone seeking weight loss in my book *The One-Day Way*. That book simplifies goals, overall fitness, and sustainable weight loss to a committed focus on what you do today. By doing the right things for just one day and then repeating them when another day arrives, you can achieve the results you've been seeking.

Now, in *Love Food and Live Well*, we are going to take the steps that will free you from the most damaging food traps. I will expose the lies that trap dieters in self-defeating habits, and I'll show you how to break free from destructive attitudes toward food. Best of all, I'll show you that fitness and weight loss don't require you to hate food. Nor do they limit you to eating only boring, bland, unsatisfying meals for the rest of your life.

This book will open your eyes to a new way of maintaining your weight, health, and fitness. We will explore healthy eating and new exercises, to be sure. And we'll arrive at the place where you will achieve all your goals and know how to maintain them for a lifetime. But what good is it to work and sweat to lose weight and get healthy if it means drudgery for the rest of your life? If it means you might extend your life span but hate every minute of it? Or if it means you live in a state of constant fear that you'll slide back into your previous self-defeating habits? Who wants that?

That's why I'm so excited about sharing the best deal you've been offered in a long, long time. Being fit and healthy doesn't require that you starve yourself or even that you hate food. It doesn't demand that you become paranoid that you'll slip up and overindulge. Nor does it require you to drag around an exercise bike every time you leave town so you can be sure to burn off the calories from that meal you enjoyed with your friends while on vacation.

The deal we're going to talk about involves more than just losing weight and getting strong and then maintaining a healthy weight for a lifetime. The deal we'll explore involves losing weight, getting strong, living healthy, and loving every minute of it. Even better, it involves loving food while we live well! Great news! We can do both of these at the same time!

We all want to enjoy life and be healthy in all areas: body, mind, and spirit, right? Plus, who wants to go through life regarding food as the enemy? God gave us food not only to keep us strong and vital but also to enjoy. That's part of the deal of a lifetime, but I'm getting ahead of myself.

———

When you're stuck in New York City, you can either shop or work. And out of desperation to meet my deadline, I chose the option that wasn't my first inclination. But I'm glad I had to stay over, because my improvised work station inspires me to tell you about the deal of a lifetime.

Soon after I sat down on this bench in sight of Wall Street, I realized this was the perfect place. Megadeals are made in this financial mecca every day. As governments and heads of state try to decide how to plug their leaking economies, I am preparing to introduce you to a deal you won't believe!

This deal is personal for you and me both. Together, we are going to find the solution to physical, emotional, and spiritual bankruptcy. Struggling with your weight, your body image, your self-confidence, and your health can exhaust and defeat you. But I am here to tell you that you can overcome the forces that want to keep you locked in a lifestyle of discouragement, failure, and despair.

The road we will take is a superhighway to claiming the life you desire, and the bonus is that you will enjoy what it takes to get there. This road is fashioned with freedom. Traveling on it, you will find the enjoyment of living well in every area of your life and experience more love than you have ever known.

When I woke up yesterday, I looked forward to getting home to hug my family the night before my daughter Ashley's first big school dance. I wasn't going to miss this for anything. I showed up at the airport nearly two hours early, which is totally not like me. I run late regularly and also miss airplanes on occasion. But not this time. I was excited and ready to get back to the zoo I call Home Sweet Home.

Ashley would be dressing up for her first homecoming dance. Jake would be an honored guest at a sports banquet where he would receive a football trophy. I was looking forward to both of these big events. Mostly, I was ready to just be Mom. You know, the lady who enjoys embarrassing her children by taking a million pictures.

As I strolled into LaGuardia Airport with time to spare, the place was in chaos. Battles were taking place everywhere, with people screaming at any airline employee in sight. I actually felt sorry for a few of them—until I had to stop and pray not to lose my cool with an insensitive airline employee myself.

I witnessed a fellow passenger sobbing uncontrollably. Between whimpers, she told the airline representative she needed to get to the wedding of her baby sister. In spite of her tears, he told her, "You should have planned better," insinuating that she should have left a few days in advance. I wanted to take him out!

But I took the route of nonviolence and tried to focus on my own flight plans. As it turned out, the woman who was about to miss her sister's wedding wasn't alone. I was about to join her with my own travel crisis. Due to bad weather, all flights to Fort Lauderdale were canceled for the night. "So sad, too bad" should be the motto of the airline industry. I was totally stuck and completely frustrated, and there seemed to be no one around who cared to find a solution. Here's a quote from the man behind the counter: "Mrs. Hobbs, we are sorry. Feel free to try us again tomorrow or perhaps the next day. It's your call."

I had to regroup and make a plan or else cry. I just went for it and did both. I needed a hotel at least for that night, so I grabbed my laptop and played a game I had played before. The Priceline.com Game, I call it. It can be fun because of the potential for saving money on a nice hotel room. Then there is an added edge of excitement that comes from the uncertainty of where you can end up for the night. I enjoy an occasional calculated risk, so I gave it a try.

First, I chose an area in New York City where I would be willing to stay. I actually put in seven. Then I decided on the quality level of the hotel. I chose four stars. (I was traveling alone in Manhattan, so safety was a factor.) Next I had to determine the price; I decided $150. This is about one-third of the going rate for a luxury hotel in this town. Then I clicked Buy and prayed. My fleece was out there, my cry was heard, and my bid was accepted! The winning hotel was in the financial district and rather swanky, judging by the name of it.

I grabbed a cab, and very soon it was obvious that the driver was lost, which is not that unusual, considering that cabbies get paid according to the meter. I phoned the hotel, and, shockingly, the front desk manager and a valet walked a full city block to find me. They also helped with my luggage. I had never been met by this kind of welcome committee in New York City. I was ecstatic. Remember, it had been a long day.

I settled into this beautiful hotel on a crisp, fall evening in the Big Apple, and then God provided one more treat. This was His way of reminding me I was under His wing for the night. Please, friends, don't laugh. I really am being completely serious. I spotted a create-a-salad establishment across the street! I went over, grabbed dinner, returned to my room, got some sleep, and then woke up inspired to write. I had the entire day to work until I would be flying home.

———

Now as I'm talking with you, sitting here bundled up in three layers of sweaters with my laptop resting on a crossed leg, I'm going to tell you about a deal that will blow away every deal made on these streets of international finance. And I'm convinced God brought me here to think about how to introduce you to the deal of a lifetime. This deal will guarantee your freedom to live well forever! I promise you, this is more real than anything I have ever known.

With the title *Love Food and Live Well*, you may be thinking this book will relate only to your relationship with food. Truthfully, it was the starting place for me when I decided to live healthy and then lost two hundred pounds. However, what I learned after I lost the weight and worked so hard to maintain it is this: after you succeed, you still face a struggle. How do you hold on to fitness and health and remain at a healthy weight without becoming obsessive about it? What good does it do to get healthy if you can't also have a life?

If you think losing two hundred pounds is hard, try losing that much weight and then learning how to enjoy life again. It's not as easy as it might sound.

But I learned that living well while loving food is entirely possible. Not only that, but feeling free to admit I like food was bigger than anything I could have imagined. It's bigger because of the word *love* attached to it. A word we often use and abuse and don't completely understand. Yet we still seek to know more about it and have more of it than anything on the planet.

Too many of us confuse love with control. In the past, most things I really loved I loved poorly. I know this because as I tried to control them, I always felt out of control. Whether it was food, friendships, jobs, or material stuff, I lived in fear—the fear of losing whatever I was trying to possess. Eventually my attempts to control everything always backfired.

My lifelong weight struggle was a perfect example. The more I made food something to control, the more weight I gained. It seems crazy, but you may be able to relate after many years of living in this tug of war. God whispered my name, and I finally answered. It was there I began a journey to freedom. Of course the release from my weight problem took time, tears, and lots of hard work. However, I realized some amazing truths along the way.

Each of us is meant to love all the things God has provided. The problem occurs when we try to cut a deal that allows us to love them on our own terms. It's tempting to try to swing a special side deal just for us so we can love food, for example, on our terms. If the deal has been designed by you, me, or the world, I can guarantee this: it will eventually lead to heartache. By seeking to maintain control, which usually involves shutting out others and propping up a false version of ourselves, who wins? Not me or you or anyone you care about, and mostly not God.

In this book I want you to recognize the power of being vulnerable. When you learn how to say, "I'm falling apart," or admit you haven't figured it all out, you can finally discover the path to peaceful living. Let's face it: you're not in control. It's healthy to admit that to yourself and to others.

Even after admitting it, it's easy to slip back into the fantasy that we can control our lives, our circumstances, and the people and the world around us. I fell back into that trap for a few minutes when my flight was canceled and I was stranded in New York. But then I remembered what I had learned the hard way, after losing two hundred pounds but still trying to control my personal world. Admitting that you're not in control and living like you really believe it are huge! If you learn this well, it will change your life.

And all of this is captured in one word—*surrender*—which is what makes the difference. Surrender to the fact that you are not in control. Admit it. Say it out loud. Believe it. In the chapters that follow, we will talk more about the power of surrender, and together we will practice living it.

Now, who doesn't love a good deal? There's a rush of adrenaline that comes when we get something of incredible value for less cost than was expected.

For me, the more I save, the more excited I feel. Can you relate? Would you be interested in a deal that would banish the pain of struggling with food and weight issues forever? At the same time, this deal will deliver excitement and a passion for living well. This means there will be filet mignon and apple pie à la mode on occasion. Can you handle that?

What if I promised this freedom would be totally free? I'd guess you might be willing to strike the deal today. But hold on; there is a catch. This deal will still cost you something: you'll have to hand over your insecurities, your pride, your self-protective habits, and your inhibitions. The deal you will be making is the same deal I made when I realized that healthy living was only a partial reward if I wasn't also living happy and fulfilled. You can be fit and strong and still enjoy life. That's what the deal of a lifetime does for you.

Before we move to the specifics of a life-changing diet and exercise program, I strongly advise you to consult your physician first. When I created the nutrition, cardio, and strength-training portions of Love Food and Live Well—the program I'll introduce you to in this book—I worked closely with experts in medicine, nutrition, and physiology. The program is sound, but, regardless, you should see your personal physician before beginning this or any nutrition, exercise, and fitness program.

Now, I want to show you how your Creator, the God of the universe, is the ultimate Deal Maker and how you can love food and live well for a lifetime.

(Before you turn the page, I would love for you to hear the song that inspired me to write this book. Please visit www.faithfoodandfitness.com and listen to "The Way You Love Me.")

PART 1

Choose a Deal That Really Delivers

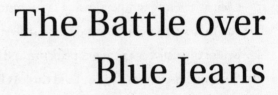

The Battle over Blue Jeans

People, Here Is My Deal!

For as long as I can remember, I have loved clothes and makeup. Even when I weighed close to 350 pounds, I experimented with trendy hairstyles while checking out the latest plus-size fashion catalogs.

When I was in elementary school, I would spend afternoons with my sister Christy, sitting on the floor of the closet in the decked-out pink bedroom we shared. This was a supersized closet where we would set up our Barbie dolls for fashion shows. Because I had blond hair and Christy was a brunette, it was only natural for me to pretend to be Barbie and her to be Skipper, Barbie's little sister. At least that's how I sold the idea to Christy. As we grew up and began to put our dolls away, I still enjoyed being prissy, often spending way too much time in front of a mirror.

Even as a young mother, I was a fashionista. I'll never forget entering the hospital to have a scheduled cesarean to deliver my son Jake. I had spent the day before the delivery getting a pedicure and manicure and shopping for a matching nightgown set. Really, I did this! As I lay on the table in the operating room, the doctor arrived and started to chuckle. "Well, Chantel, I can see nothing about this is going to be a natural delivery." All I could say was, "At least I left the false eyelashes at home." I was only half kidding.

One reason I went overboard with my appearance was because I loved hearing friends and family comment on how together I looked. Even while having a baby, I wanted to look great. But today, in hindsight, I feel seriously sorry for the woman I used to be. She was always exhausted from trying to maintain her unreal image. Plus, I knew deep down that I wasn't fooling anyone but myself. My weight problem wasn't going to vanish underneath fancy clothing and attempts to camouflage my problem areas. I really did know that owning an all-black wardrobe wouldn't keep my body issues a secret.

But back then I had convinced myself I needed to make a serious effort to look pretty from the neck up because I was too overweight for the rest of me to look decent. I rationalized that if I could highlight my best features, people would see my positive attributes and look past my greatest flaw: my obese body. At this point my life was one big head game.

I'll never forget the weekend I went on a business trip with my husband, Keith, to Bermuda. This was a dream coming true for someone who spent most days watching Barney and folding laundry. But when we started to pack, panic set in. Bermuda is one huge beach, and I knew I'd embarrass my husband if I wore a swimsuit in front of his bosses and work friends. On the other hand, this was Bermuda! It was a free trip and a chance to escape the zoo I called home!

After we boarded the plane, I found my seat and immediately put a jacket over my waist. This was a trick I had learned from previous travel experiences, and it almost always worked. If I could hide where the seat belt was supposed to be, the flight attendant wouldn't notice that mine was unbuckled. The truth is, I did this because I couldn't connect the seat belt. I was too big around. This time, however, my system failed. As the attendant stopped by our row, she asked me to buckle my seat belt. As I struggled to latch it, she stood impatiently with one hand on her hip. I whispered that I was having trouble making it fit.

So being the sensitive, tall, and freakishly thin woman she was, she shouted to her co-worker, "Could you look in one of the overhead compartments for a seat-belt extension?"

I was mortified. I closed my eyes and tried to pretend the attendant was talking about someone else. A few moments later she handed me the hated seat-belt extension, and I fastened the thing as quickly as I could. I promise you, I could feel the pity of strangers as they witnessed my shame. But instead of shedding tears, I did what I had rehearsed in previous situations. I took a deep breath and grabbed Keith's hand, squeezing it for dear life as the aircraft took off. *My vacation is off to a great start,* I told myself. *I can't wait to see what other embarrassing moments lie ahead.*

Surprisingly, our Bermuda trip ended up being the trip of a lifetime. The island was beautiful, the water was the clearest blue I had ever seen, and I felt beautiful for the entire week. Strangely, it was another young mother, the wife of one of Keith's co-workers, who was mostly responsible.

Each day I would get dolled up and make my entrance into the meeting room for the company's group breakfast. This girl went out of her way to say something sincere and extraordinary about the way I looked, morning after morning. She would also ask me for fashion advice. By her looks, she didn't need any, certainly none from me. Yet she still inquired and never in a condescending way.

Best of all, she never breathed the dreaded words "You have such a pretty face." The trip to Bermuda taught me the intense power we all have when we speak to someone, especially to a person who is feeling weak and vulnerable. Just by saying something simple and positive, we can brighten someone's outlook, even if it's only for a few seconds.

For most of my life I had become accustomed to backhanded compliments. When it came to my weight and all my failed attempts to lose it, I had heard everything. I'd try yet another diet, and two weeks into it over and over I would hear from those around me, "Now keep up the good work." And I would always think, *Are you kidding? I'm trying here. Just tell me "good job," and don't worry about whether I lose another dad-gum pound. I get that you are letting me know I have a long way to go!*

Yet Another New Start

Coming home from Bermuda, where I felt sincere acceptance, I had real hope. I felt different. I was relaxed, revived, and encouraged. I decided that I was ready to give weight loss another shot. As I set out to lose weight for the eighty-sixth time in my life, I felt prepared. I bought the latest diet book from Sam's Club and a twelve-pack of muffins. I rationalized the muffin purchase by telling myself I needed to have one last hurrah.

On Monday my plan was to go for it. I would try with everything in me not to let anything stand in my way. Of course, I didn't see any need to crack open the new book I'd bought until the weekend was over! What would a few more days of indulgence hurt?

Then Monday arrived, and I made my grand entrance at the gym. I even went back three days in a row. The only problem was that by the end of the week I was hanging out more than working out. I'd been trying to get David, the juice bar owner, to tell me his recipe for the yummy chocolate–peanut butter protein shake I was ordering every day. The first clue it wasn't all that healthy should have been the chocolate syrup he poured in. But I told myself, if it's made on gym property, how bad could it be?

By the time the week ended, I had followed the plan in my recently purchased book and had my cheat day. Not surprisingly, I quickly indulged in an entire cheat weekend. However, I managed to get back to the gym the following Monday. The plan I was on was doable, and even with halfhearted efforts, I was slowly losing weight.

After shedding about twenty pounds, I decided I needed some new clothes. This was kind of funny, especially since not one person had noticed that I had lost an ounce. As I said earlier, I've always loved fashion. But at this point, with my weight so high, I was stuck wearing mostly dresses and skirts. I just couldn't face the prospect of trying to fit my behind into a pair of pants at Lane Bryant. But now, since I was feeling pretty good about myself and getting results, I headed over to the Coral Square Mall. I was there to hunt down a pair of blue jeans. Even if I had to lie down to zip them and not breathe while I wore them, I was determined to come home with new jeans.

I picked up three pairs with plenty of stretch to take into the dressing room. Once the door was closed, though, no amount of sucking it in, squeezing hard, or holding my breath got the jeans up to my waist. I couldn't make any of them fit. As I held the jeans up and looked in the mirror, I wondered how anyone could stand to look at me. I was a disgusting blob of pain and misery.

I had left home that day feeling good about my progress. I was finally losing some weight. But after a few minutes in a dressing room, I wanted to die. How had I let myself become this pathetic mess of a woman?

A few Cinnabons later I went home. Two weeks after my blue jean horror show, I found out I was expecting. A month into the pregnancy I miscarried due to a badly infected gallbladder, and I ended up having emergency surgery. I wondered if I would ever change my life or if I would die first. Death seemed like perhaps the only escape out of this prison.

About six months later I had an unforgettable encounter with God. I was alone in my car, driving home from a meeting. I had reached my lowest point ever, and I let God in. I had known Him for years, ever since I had been saved from an eternity separated from Him. As a little girl in Sunday school, I had asked Jesus into my heart to save me from my sins. What I needed now, as a desperate, hurting, damaged woman, was to be saved from myself. I was still trying to run my own life.

God had whispered my name through many embarrassing moments and hurtful situations; I just never answered. But that night, alone in my car, He finally got through to me. I experienced a supernatural intervention. And it compels me now to tell my friends, my clients, and my readers my Lazarus story.

An Incredible Second Chance

Remember the story of Lazarus in the Bible? When Jesus brought him back from the dead, and we're talking dead as a doornail (he was four-days dead), I imagine all he wanted was to blow a trumpet and tell the world about his miracle. Today I feel a similar kind of zeal resulting from my own miracle. As I surrendered all the pain of my lifelong weight problem to God, my heart began a major shift. God gave me a deep desire to go to work. For the first time, I took on the task of losing the weight with Him in charge. I was no longer alone as I had been in the past. By allowing God, who never breaks a promise, to give me the strength, self-control, and focus I needed, how could I fail?

Ten years later I am on the same course He set for my life that night. My life is still filled with unexpected moments, both tragedies and celebrations. But I have never looked back.

After going on to lose two hundred pounds, I designed my own fitness and weight-loss program and became a certified Spinning teacher, personal trainer, and marathon runner. I love feeling strong, being healthy, and knowing I'm not a slave to my former appetites. Often I run into people I haven't seen in many years. They may have known me as the overweight girl with a pretty face. And if I dare to attempt a reacquaintance, I am usually in for a good laugh.

I'll never forget one woman from a church I attended years earlier. I ran into her at the grocery store and tried to convince her who I was. "You aren't really Chantel from West Lauderdale Baptist," she insisted. I tried to get her to believe it was me, just an improved version. I think she finally accepted the truth, but it took awhile.

I am proud of the woman I have worked to become. However, I am most thankful that God rescued me from a place where I had lost all hope. God's care for me and His work in my life give me the strength to stay on course. Now, after writing four books and producing a learning system for weight loss and fitness, I can see that God continues to use me as a voice of real-life experience. A big part of my message is this: let me help you stop sabotaging yourself and your life. I know, from hard experience, how to overcome self-defeat. Every day I get to hear the stories of people who were losing hope, as I was, and now are finding the life they had dreamed of. I receive e-mails from women who have heard me speak, read one of my books, or heard me on the radio and now are surrendering their failed attempts to God. They are learning the truth and power of surrender and then doing the hard work of changing their lives.

In my work of helping people reclaim their health, I never know what is coming next. Recently I got a call from my publicist. She was so excited she could hardly tell me the news. "While you are in New York later this week to do *The Today Show* and *Fox and Friends,* a major women's magazine wants to set up a photo shoot."

I screamed. I couldn't help it. Not only would the exposure help sell my book, but doing a photo shoot in New York, as the author of fitness books, was an experience I never dreamed I'd have. When I weighed nearly 350 pounds, an opportunity like this never entered my mind.

I couldn't wait, but I had to. It was still a few weeks away. As New Year's came and went, I was more careful than ever about fitting in all my workouts and eating clean. (*Clean eating* is the best way for me to think about food that delivers maximum energy with a reasonable calorie content.) When the day arrived, a driver came to our New York hotel to take Keith and me to the shoot. In the previous week, I had given my measurements to a stylist. She informed me she would be shopping for the clothes I would wear for the photo shoot. To use a term from my Southern-rooted parents, I was in hog heaven! I used to be the woman who was embarrassed to tell anyone her sizes, and now I had someone else buying me clothes based on them! The great part was the freedom in sharing what size I was. For the first time, I felt no shame.

When we arrived at the studio, I noticed that the loft where the photographer had scheduled the shoot was trendy and chic. It had sky-high ceilings complete with lots of lights and screened umbrellas to ensure perfect lighting. Taking up an entire wall was a buffet of food the magazine had catered for the event, my event! All of it was healthy fare with me in mind.

As I entered a dressing room, fun music filled the air. A makeup artist and hairstylist began their magic. I listened while they talked about their past work. One had done Heidi Klum's makeup not long before, and the other spoke of doing the makeup for big names on a major movie set. I was a little overwhelmed with the emotion of the moment. I felt like I was back to playing Barbie dolls with my sister.

After hair and makeup were underway, the stylist had me try on all the clothes she had bought. We settled on a great pair of designer jeans with a sleek white sweater and a trendy hot pink top. I put on the heels she had purchased—a perfect fit—and some fabulous jewelry. Then I was whisked away to the main part of the studio. In that moment I felt like a million bucks.

It was then the stylist asked me what I believed to be an insane question: "Where are your old blue jeans?" At first I couldn't believe I had heard her right, but I knew what she was getting at. She said the creative director wanted me to hold up a supersized pair of pants in the photo to show the dramatic contrast represented by clothes I had worn in my previous life.

I understood the point of playing up the shock value. Shoppers standing in line at the supermarket checkout would be amazed by the pants I had once filled out. But the idea that I would have to display a symbol of the old life I had left behind made me feel sick, like I had never lost a pound. How could I hold up a pair of jeans that represented my old humiliation?

I explained to the stylist that not only had I not brought a pair of jeans but I didn't feel comfortable doing this. As I held my breath, a few phone calls were made, and the shoot continued without the troubling reminder of my past. It turned out to be a great experience, and I was pleased with the photographs. However, I felt a little angry and upset with myself. Hadn't I moved on past my old image? I could now fit two of me inside my old jeans, so why was this such a big deal? I also wondered if readers might have been helped by seeing me holding up the pants I used to wear. Why couldn't I just smile into the camera with confidence even if I was standing behind a pair of my old jeans?

I WILL NEVER RETURN

Back in my hotel room, I awoke in the middle of the night still thinking about the photo shoot. Finally I could see clearly what had offended me. Supersized blue jeans were a symbol of major pain in my life. Holding them up in front of me would not feel as if I was showcasing success. I was now on an exciting journey to share my life and my program to help other people. I had ditched the old jeans, just as I had ditched diets—and both of them for good! Sure, I will always be able to relate to the woman who desperately tries to zip up a pair of pants in a store's dressing room. But I didn't want to spend another special moment of my life sharing the spotlight with my former self. I had crossed the point of no return. I now knew without question that I would never go back.

I have a completely new deal, one that focuses on living my new life, the life that God led me to when I fell into my darkest moment. The old me had long wanted to leave behind the constant torment of being overweight and undisciplined. That life is now over. My new deal is much sweeter than I dreamed was possible.

You can have the same deal! You can start living a life of security and freedom. You can be released from the prison of defeat, failure, and negative self-image. And best of all, the new deal we're going to explore is guaranteed to last.

I won't ever return to being the person I started out as. There is no going back. And I'll show you how to take full advantage of the same deal!

Want Chocolate? You've Got a Deal!

Learn How to Love Food and Still Live Well

I receive e-mails from a lot of people who have read my earlier books, and I'm convinced many of the readers typed through teary eyes. I even meet struggling women when I'm running errands and when I travel. Many times I have listened to a new friend pour out her heart while seated next to me on a flight or standing in the grocery store checkout line with small children hanging on to her.

When it comes to coping with food, most people I know—even those who have done a great job of losing weight—still feel overwhelmed. No matter how much they have worked on their food issues, food is still the enemy in their eyes. Losing weight may be the initial battle, but it is not the real war. Keeping the weight off without losing our sanity is the far greater challenge—the big kahuna of life.

How to Win the Fitness War and Identify the Real Enemy

You can't win a war if you haven't identified the true enemy. First, food is not the enemy. Before you reject this idea and skip to the next chapter, hear me out. The real opposition is never the obvious thing. For example, your enemy is not the intoxicating aroma of popcorn at a movie theater. It isn't even the hot-out-of-the-oven bread that is set in front of you at a steakhouse, complete with real butter to tantalize you.

Sure, food is a challenge. But every one of us has been fighting a more troublesome opponent: ourselves! Our skewed thinking and mixed-up brains are the culprits. We defeat ourselves in advance by the way we rig our minds to think about food. For too long we have believed that the biggest and hardest struggle we face is the raw desire to eat the foods we crave. Then, if we give in, we tell ourselves that we are weak and lacking in self-discipline. This combination is the most effective way to defeat yourself and sabotage your health and fitness.

Some people have convinced themselves that gaining and losing weight like a yo-yo is their destiny. Come on, friends. Isn't it ridiculous to think anyone is destined to fail after achieving a great victory? It is not your destiny to go through life with low self-worth. It is always wrong to define yourself as a failure. I don't buy it, and you shouldn't either.

My past struggles with food came from the battles that were going on in my head. Even after I lost two hundred pounds and was working as a Spinning instructor, I still had to deal with how I saw myself. Can you relate to this struggle? Perhaps you have achieved incredible goals and still wonder, deep inside, if you really are a failure.

IT'S TIME TO CLAIM YOUR NEW IDENTITY

If you share this struggle, allow the truth in this chapter to set you free. The title of this book promises that you can love food and live well. But what do you think it means to love food? Do you think it would be a bad thing for you to scream out in the shower, "I love food!"? You might frighten the kids, but it's not wrong to love food. So as we gain an accurate understanding of ourselves, the role of food, and the meaning of love, you will abandon your former approach to loving food. And especially if you have lost weight recently, it's time to let go of your old habits and past self-identity.

Hear me out. For years I loved food with reckless abandon—and on a regular basis. This was back in the heyday of my weight problem, when my hangouts were bakeries and barbecue restaurants. If you have ever struggled with food issues, I guarantee that your life will be transformed when you gain a healthy approach to loving food. Shouting "I love food" and not feeling guilty is liberating. Go ahead, give it a try.

The Bible says, "Perfect love casts out fear" (1 John 4:18), which means love and fear can't coexist. Aren't you tired of fearing food, your perceived enemy, and thinking that any moment your behind will grow wider if you speak the words, "I love warm chocolate-chip cookies with a glass of cold milk?" It's time we put food in perspective, rethink our identity, and then love ourselves and food in a way that contributes to health and fitness.

My previous way of loving food was an unhealthy obsession. By pondering all the choices available at most meals, I'd often choose an entrée with the belief that it would fill my need for happiness and control. And every time I chose to eat something, I would feel in control and happy—for about five seconds. Just until the next time I walked past a mirror and realized that I was wearing my control issues.

Here is the full truth: God never intended for us to be entirely in control. My efforts to exert control locked me inside a prison. I thank God I am now free from that. And having enjoyed freedom for ten years, I realize that the key to being set free was to redefine love.

I grew up in a loving home, and I married a man who loves me without placing conditions on my appearance. My children are great, I have great friends, and still I was confused about love. I think that's true for a lot of us, because the word *love* is tricky to figure out. Is it a feeling or an action, something that comes unexpectedly out of nowhere or something we work on and develop over time? No matter how you define love, I know that it feels good to love and be in love. And since most of us struggle with food and the things we believe it does to us (related to weight, health, and appetites), you and I are going to get to the bottom of this issue.

Here is my promise to you: I will show you that we can love food and still maintain a healthy weight, without going out of our minds. For nearly everyone who has lost weight through dieting and then put the weight back on, one of three things has been true. Either they loved food in a way that led to weight gain, or they denied their love of food and it drove them crazy, or they loved food and gained weight and lived in denial.

We're going to overcome all three by doing something completely new. We will develop a love of food, maintain a healthy weight, and stay sane. Are you ready?

LOVE FOOD AND LIVE WELL

This is not an impossible dream. I know because I have achieved it, and I have helped others to do the same thing. It can be your reality too, if you want it. I can truthfully say I love all kinds of food. And most food, I really, really, really love! However, my definition of the love I have for food is not the same one I had when I was overweight.

To make this transition, I had to develop a completely new thought process. It started working after I broke it down into its components:

- What is the real role of food?
- How can I love food and choose well without being controlled and then defeated by guilt?

Both of these are essential. You have to get real about food and the role it plays in your life—not just in physical survival but in your mind, your emotions, and your lifestyle. Equally important is to let go of any guilt that still lingers. You can't move on until you do this. The guilt will drive you crazy, and you'll find yourself doing things like trying to pinpoint the voice of the little devil on your shoulder who's whispering in your ear, "Go ahead and eat the second piece of cake. It's sooo good." You may even allow guilt to push you to beat yourself up by skipping the next three meals as payback for eating some extra cake.

Forget this old mentality, and replace it with truth and reality. The cake was good! You knew it after the first few bites. And if you had stopped eating it sooner, you still would have known how good it tasted. But—and this is important—if you had stopped eating it, you would also have skipped the regret! Regret will drag you down and sap your strength. You don't need it, so let go of it. You need to abandon all the memories of poor choices you have made. Like perhaps the time you went slightly crazy and ate your entire Cobb salad and then your kids' french fries and chicken nuggets. You didn't want to waste food—at least that's what you told yourself (knowing McDonald's doesn't recycle the scraps and ship them overseas).

Or is there a day in your past that you need to let go of—the day you consumed an entire box of Samoa cookies while thinking, *All I'm really doing is supporting the Girl Scout troop*? You might have then bought two more boxes and made them your breakfast and lunch for the entire week. You have to let go of those days and delete them from your memory. If you can't let go of regret over past missteps, you can't receive the truth, and only truth will free you from guilt, self-judgment, low self-worth, and the yo-yo dieting that most of us are way too familiar with.

What I'm about to tell you is not only the truth. It definitely works! Very soon you will enjoy ordering dessert without feeling as if you're being bad. Food will no longer control you as it has in the past. Isn't truth a lot more attractive when it not only puts a spotlight on the lies you believe but also improves your life and helps you achieve your goals?

Think about people you know who are naturally thin, some you may even have to work hard not to hate. They can eat a big meal whenever they want to without feeling guilty. They don't waste time obsessing about what they ate last week or three months ago. Once I learned how to do this myself, I knew I would never go back to my former defeated, guilt-ridden way of living.

After I lost two hundred pounds, it seemed like only a few seconds before everyone I had met since birth started coming to me for advice about their food issues—as if I didn't still have my own issues! Here I was, trying to figure out how to reach a goal weight I could live with and not gain any back, and suddenly others thought of me as an expert.

Initially I was hesitant to give advice. As time went by, though, I listened to the struggles of others and offered encouragement, which helped keep me focused. That's the beauty of sharing our struggles and victories.

BEATING THE SCARCITY LIE

One girlfriend I have known forever, who has waged her own weight war, called me not long ago. "Chantel, why is it when someone offers me a candy bar, I look at it as if this is the very last time I will be given the opportunity to eat one?" I knew exactly what she meant. My friend had identified one of the biggest lies that continue to defeat us. Instead of eating foods we especially like at an appropriate time, we get the idea there might not ever be another chance to indulge.

But think about this: if you knew in advance the time and date you would next eat a steak or dessert or whatever your favorite food is, then it would be no great feat to resist the temptation. It would be much easier today to say good-bye to a candy bar, knowing you'd be saying hello to a banana split that you'd make with the kids on Friday night. I believe it's the "not knowing when" that makes us think we'd better indulge now because this might be our last chance.

The only thing this last-chance mind-set guarantees is that you're forfeiting your last chance to maintain a healthy weight. So once I reached my sustainable weight, I set out to plan a weight-maintenance program that dispels the lie of scarcity. The theory in a nutshell is this: my favorite foods are not scarce, and there is an appropriate time to celebrate with them. Because I love a candy bar on occasion, I wanted the freedom to say it without guilt or shame: "I love a candy bar every now and then."

To prove my theory and gain some insight, I interviewed people, but not just anyone. I searched for the leanest of the pack, the forever-fit women who enjoy all-fruit smoothies and never gain an ounce. In my mind they had to be freaks of nature. How could they not be gaining back the weight?

But when I interviewed them, I learned a lesson to last a lifetime! I cornered Becky one day in the gym. I was supercasual, so she had no idea I was interviewing her. Becky is thin and fit, way more fit than I will ever be. She is so fit, in fact, that one time I watched her run fifteen miles on a treadmill and then dab a few drops of sweat, throw on a T-shirt, and head out for the day. To put this into perspective, when I run five miles on a treadmill, other gym patrons have occasionally handed me wads of paper towels. They are pretty sure my beach towel won't suffice. When I run, I think people are convinced I'm trying to escape someone who's chasing me with a knife!

Thin-and-fit Becky is the kind of woman you try to hate. She has never, not even for a day, experienced pain due to her weight. So she isn't insecure about how she looks. That makes you want to hate her even more, but you can't because she is so sweet.

I started the interview by asking about a past pregnancy and how her body had responded. "Well, I started out at about 118 pounds and then ballooned up to 143 pounds!" *Gasp! You were out of control,* I joked silently. "Then I had the baby and started breast-feeding, and the weight just seemed to fall off." I tried to hate her a little, but I couldn't. She was too matter-of-fact.

Then she explained that as her life became more hectic, caring for a newborn, she would forget to eat. So she also had the headache of trying to gain weight. Breast-feeding was really melting off the pounds.

I asked, "Do you eat whatever you want?" And wouldn't you know it, she said yes. I joked, "Sure you do, as long as it's green, leafy, and marked organic, right?" That's when she told me how much she loves chocolate. She said she eats chocolate every day! Now my ears began to perk up. Could this really be true? Could someone really eat chocolate regularly and look this good? I had to know more.

So I said, "Tell me about your day, what you eat, where you go, what you do." I mean, inquiring minds want to know.

"Well, I get up early," Becky said, "and after I get the kids off to school, I exercise for an hour. Immediately I have breakfast. I'm starving by then, and it's about 8:30. I have either a protein shake or oatmeal and eggs, sometimes cereal. I do household chores and grab a banana and almonds. At lunch I eat a sandwich and pretzels or baked chips. Occasionally I have a cookie. I also love biscotti and tea.

"When the kids get home, I do homework with them and have my treat. It's usually a few pieces of Dove chocolate or frozen yogurt with granola on top. And dinner is somewhat simple: grilled chicken and veggies or a salad and sweet potatoes. And I love rice and black beans. They are my favorite."

I actually gasped. How could this tiny woman put away so much food and still be this tiny woman?

"So you're telling me that you have a treat every day, but for the majority of the day you try to eat light and healthy?" Then she explained what became, for me, the eureka moment!

"I don't think of it that way," she said. "I just have the same food most days and don't deny myself something if I really want it."

I had one question left: "So would you consider eating the entire bag of Dove chocolates at once?"

(Get ready for the eureka moment.)

She said: "If I did, then there wouldn't be any left for tomorrow!"

So there you have it, folks. Becky has been "watching it" for so long she doesn't even consider herself to be watching it. This is where I want to live: in this Oz with Becky and other thin, strong, fit women. I want to be a strong, healthy, fit woman who lives comfortably in a world that is dripping with chocolate and laced with frozen treats. I want to approach food in a way that leaves me full of anticipation of the next day's delights! And at the same time, I would be free from the feeling that today is the last day I'll ever be able to enjoy something delicious.

I need you to pay attention closely if you want the same thing. If you love food in the right way today, you can love food again tomorrow and also the day after that. There is no scarcity of good things, so you don't have to over-indulge, fearing that this will be your last chance to enjoy food.

THE BEST WAY TO LOVE FOOD

Without knowing it, Becky introduced me to a new way to live and a new way to think about food. First, loving food is not a sin. How could it be? God gave us the ability to taste. He wants us to have this enjoyment in life. It is a God-given source of pleasure. The problems arise when we take something that's good and allow its pleasure to become so addictive that we stop practicing self-control and regular restraint.

I have seen people struggle in the same way with golf, the desire for expensive clothes or homes, drugs, sex, and, *ouch*, even exercise! God wants us to serve only one Master: Him. Serving anything or anyone else to the point of compulsion always causes misery and pain. The love itself isn't the problem; it's the mistake of loving obsessively and directing that intense love toward the wrong object—in this case, food. Love that we fail to limit and control causes pain and agony. I love my husband, but if he were to ask me to rob a bank with him, sorry, babe, I'm staying home. The love is still there, but I can't risk dishonoring God in order to follow my husband. The same is true with food issues. The love is appropriate, because God gave us food and the ability to enjoy it, and we need it for survival. However, if our love for food causes us to be fat, we must check the motives of our heart. If carrying too much weight is your deal or if you're letting food consume your thought life, it's time to do some pruning.

Just as an orchard owner prunes the fruit trees to keep them healthy so they'll produce more fruit, it's healthy for us to prune aspects of our lives. Here is how it applies to regrowing a healthy love relationship with food. First, you'll need to let go of your love for food for a season. If done in the right way, your love for it will regrow in a healthy, God-ordained way. That's why in my first book, *Never Say Diet*, I teach people how to willingly sacrifice favorite foods and explain why food should be boring. When you temporarily set aside your love of food, use the time and the new experience to search your heart. Ask yourself an important question: what is my deal as it relates to food, body image, self-image, and what I believe about my destiny? We all struggle with big things that affect our lives more than we like to admit. So what's your deal? Think about it.

In the chapters to come, we will learn about a healthy body image, try some recipes, and practice principles for celebrating with food. I will also introduce new and fun exercises. However, before you move on, figure out what your deal is. It could take a few minutes or a few hours or a few days. Take as much time as you need, but don't skip over it.

The Power of Surrender

When I was morbidly obese, I found that many people wanted me to be in control. I shared the same desire. I wanted to control my life, my weight, my future—everything! Yet I finally had to accept reality, which is that none of us can ever be fully in control. Allowing God to take control is the only way to live that makes everything else fall into place. When I realized this, I began to experience true liberty.

God whispered my name on the night I cried out to Him. That is when my heart shifted and my weight-loss journey began. It was the beginning of a new life. I decided that night, in prayer, that I had to stop trying to run the show. Finally grasping God's love for me, I would never go down the old road again. I surrendered to God that night, and that changed my life.

Have you decided that you won't go back down your old road? I know it's not easy to once and for all decide you are leaving your old life behind. It creates uncertainty, and you lose familiar habits and ways of doing things. It leads you into the unknown.

But you don't have to go there alone. That's why I'm here. Deciding to change your life doesn't put an end to temptation. You won't suddenly solve your food issues or get your eating habits under control. But when you find yourself struggling, you can pray for strength. That's what I did and still do. Whenever I feel I'm veering toward the exit ramp, I remind myself that the new road I've chosen leads to health and a good self-image, whereas the road I used to be on led to a cliff.

Changing your life begins with your mind. You must decide that you are done with trying and failing, losing weight and then gaining it back, setting goals for a healthy life and then falling back into old habits. First you change your mind, and then you can change your body and your life. If you desire to live in freedom for the rest of your life, you must shift your thinking. You have to ditch the diet mentality of deprivation.

You have reached a crossroads where you can choose to change your life for good. If you are ready, welcome! Your deal is about to mesh with the God of the universe. And does He have a deal for you!

The Barbie Myth Is the World's Deal

Don't Buy the Lie—None of Us Can Afford It

In 1959 little girls everywhere were introduced to a new friend. She measured just eleven and a half inches tall, but you would never know it by the bigness of what she stands for today, more than fifty years later. She is said to be the picture of perfection, and her name is Barbie. Sure, she's only a doll, a mere toy. But there is a bigger reason she has stood the test of time.

Her creator, Ruth Handler, designed Barbie with greater dreams in mind. In her autobiography Handler shares her desire for little girls to "have an outlet to enhance self-image, and a way to expand their sense of potential."[1] The thought was a noble one: to help girls consider greater possibilities for their lives. But it's a lot of pressure to put on a piece of plastic poured into a mold. All in all, I would say that Barbie has displayed her own dreams quite well.

An academic once calculated the odds of an actual woman being shaped like Barbie. Fewer than one in one hundred thousand women were found to have a body that approximated the doll's dimensions. But even with her outlandish and unrealistic proportions, Barbie has no trouble attracting new fans. Perhaps it's due to her frequent shifts in identity. Just when you think you have her figured out, she switches careers or gets a new luxurious home. Over the years she has been a dentist, doctor, astronaut, and paleontologist. Long before there was Sarah Palin, there was Barbie. She even ran for president in the 1990s. And no matter what fast-paced lifestyle she adopts, she always looks stress free. She lives in a dream house, vacations in a high-tech mobile home, and owns a loft apartment in the city and a yacht. Barbie has interests in many businesses, from hair salons to bakeries. And, of course, the voluptuous doll has a figure for girls everywhere to envy.

But what effect has this fifty-year-old toy really had on girls and their self-image? Has it been dangerous or delightful? Mattel, the manufacturer, reported revenues of $4.7 billion from sales of the doll in 2000. The average girl between the ages of three and eleven owns ten of them. Barbie is sold in more than 150 countries.[2]

Sadly, the doll that approximates fewer than one in one hundred thousand women now represents the world's deal. And I believe it's a deal you want to avoid—and you want your daughters to avoid.

PERFECTION IS NOT REAL

According to one scientist, if Barbie were life-size, she'd stand five feet nine inches tall and weigh 110 pounds. Guess you could say she has no meat on her bones. If she went to see her primary-care doctor, he'd inquire if she was suffering from an eating disorder. His reasoning? Stats show one out of four women do. And if a woman is five nine and weighs only 110 pounds, she's in trouble. Of course, Barbie would deny it, explaining that she eats an orange and some apples every day. She might forget to mention that she also sneaks a 100-calorie bag of popcorn. But that's pretty much it!

Barbie's human weight would reach only 76 percent of what is considered a healthy weight for a woman of her height. (She falls short by nearly forty pounds.) Plus, if she were human, she would have to walk on all fours due to the drastic proportions of her arms, legs, and torso. Her measurements, were she human, would be 39-18-33. Likely she has no healthy body fat. Therefore, she wouldn't menstruate. This pretty much destroys her chances of getting pregnant. (Not to mention she's now past fifty.)

I feel sorry for this woman. Trying not to look a day over nineteen for the past fifty years seems like it would be exhausting—and expensive. She also faces the added pressure of fitting into the ever-expanding wardrobe she is provided. Her fashions look like they came straight off the runway. Recently, elementary school–age girls have begun dressing their Barbies in lingerie as well. This must be slightly uncomfortable for her.

I imagine Barbie walking into a meeting with the folks who design her clothes. She begins by batting her brilliant blue eyes. Then she begs for leeway on the next collection. "Please stop making jeans so low-rise." The trendy fashions make her uncomfortable. She's convinced the designers don't take into account she is practically entering menopause, which makes her fight a thickening midsection. All the Pilates and Spin classes in the world can't reverse nature. Barbie has to constantly watch herself.

And there are the nightly backaches. She has to keep a heating pad by her bed. Carrying those enormous breasts on her small frame takes its toll. She even has a permanent bra-strap dent on her shoulders.

Then there's the matter of her bleached-blond locks and keeping up with the dark roots. Having perfect hair is a job in itself. She must visit her hairdresser every two weeks. One great thing is that she can get her teeth whitened at the mall, where there is a kiosk for just about everything. It's perfect, since Starbucks is also in the mall. This is where Barbie and her less-attractive friend Teresa can meet for coffee and gossip. Getting manicures and pedicures, having eyebrows waxed, going for facials—it's all necessary for her to keep being Barbie. And let's not forget the false eyelashes, lip plumper, and lunch-hour Botox visits. If you have ever envied a magazine-cover model and tried to mimic her look, you understand the intense pressure.

Finally, she has to run a household with all the cooking, cleaning, and laundry. Barbie also cares for her husband, Ken. (What does he do all day, anyway?) With so many job titles for this wonder woman and so much pressure from the media, this girl needs serious prayer. (Really, all of us girls need serious prayer.) But without prayer, our imagined human version of Barbie is at risk of a nervous breakdown. She is a prime candidate to end up in rehab. Although Straitjacket Barbie would be a strange addition to the line, at least she would be more realistic.

THE SERIOUS SIDE OF THE SILLINESS

It's exhausting to keep up an image. The media have sought to make us slaves to beauty, dieting, mirror gazing, and self-absorption. Whose thin is in? In the 1960s it was Twiggy, a willowy version of Kate Moss. Both of these women appear so thin in photographs that it's frightening. They represent someone's idea of beauty, but it's not a realistic view.

We know it hasn't always been this way. If you enjoy watching old movies, you have seen robust women from the 1950s, such as Sophia Loren, Marilyn Monroe, and Jane Russell. They were voluptuous, beautiful, glamorous women who defined feminine beauty. So what's going on? What is the world's deal when it comes to our bodies?

Advertisers continue to taunt us with magazines at the checkout stand meant to mess with our minds. Sure, the faces are different, but the message never changes. The media pretend to answer the very question they have the nerve to pose in the first place. Cover blurbs such as "Are You Happy with Your Fuller Figure?" have the power to wreak havoc on a woman who is feeling down on herself. Am I thin enough, like Jennifer Aniston? Can I have skin and lips like Angelina Jolie and still keep up with my children? After all, she has like a hundred of them to keep up with and still looks red-carpet gorgeous. I read a magazine cover recently with a real kicker for anyone struggling with body image: "How you can get your body back, like singer and mom Faith Hill." Are you joking me? Please, someone remind me—on what day did Faith lose her great body?

A study conducted at the University of Missouri–Columbia found something even more alarming. After eighty-one young women studied a standard fashion magazine cover to cover, all eighty-one said they felt worse about themselves.[3] These findings are troubling but, sadly, not surprising. What does the world's deal teach us? First, we don't measure up. Second, unless we look like the glamorous women on the magazine covers, we're inferior. It's time we stop accepting the world's deal, because it's a rotten one.

Hollywood works overtime to redefine the look that is "normal" and to give us unrealistic goals for what a healthy body weight should be. I want to know what happened to the attractiveness of childbearing hips or simply looking good for your man. I'm convinced many women are trying harder to impress other women than they are their personal love interest. The truth is that only a small fraction of women possess the genetic makeup to achieve an ultralong and ultrathin body. So why is this exceedingly rare body type continually presented as the ideal? The honest answer is that it's done to keep us frustrated and believing that we need them for help and answers. It feeds several multibillion-dollar industries.

A study called "About-Face" found that twenty-five years ago the average female fashion model weighed only 8 percent less than the average woman. Currently, the average female model weighs 23 percent less than the average woman.[4] With magazine covers everywhere you turn, plus the Internet, movies, and television, it's no shock that women feel inadequate and dissatisfied with their looks.

Here is the real kicker: over the course of the last twenty years, women who don't earn their living as models have become heavier! All the while, the images of beauty that they see have become thinner and leaner. Can you say, "Emotional overeating"? In other words, if you can't join 'em, you might as well eat up to cheer up.

FEARING FOR OUR DAUGHTERS

I recall reading a few years ago about an actress from a popular sitcom who had battled a terrible flu for nearly a month. By the time she came back to the studio set, she had lost about fifteen pounds. She was nervous about going back to work because she knew her eyes looked dark and sunken and her face was emaciated. Even her size 4 jeans were loose and hanging on her. Feeling self-conscious, she quietly went into wardrobe and makeup. When people saw her, there was a stir. Men and women came in to congratulate her on the weight loss.

Do you see the craziness of this? The actress had lost weight as the result of an illness. She felt terrible about the way she looked, and people were congratulating her!

This went on all day. People were begging to know the secret to her weight loss. She responded that she had been near death with the flu, and she will never forget one response in particular. It was, basically, "Whatever you got, give it to me. It sure is working for you."

She was shocked, wondering if she had heard correctly. Not one person asked how she was feeling. Instead, it was more like, "Wow, girl, you really wear sickness well!"

The actress told this story to encourage young women to be aware of the messages they are receiving and to make the point that our priorities no longer bend toward wellness. Instead, the messages that assault us are twisted into a trap, telling us to do whatever it takes to be thinner. Even if it means embracing illness!

People, we need to wake up. If we don't, we'll never be able to shut out the lies and protect ourselves from body-image madness. A recent poll of girls in high school revealed disturbing findings, which were presented in a congressional briefing. "These girls said they were more afraid of becoming fat than they are of nuclear war, cancer, or losing their parents."[5] And apparently 71 percent of adolescent girls want to be thinner despite only a small proportion of them exceeding a healthy weight.[6]

I also read that by age thirteen, 53 percent of American girls are "unhappy with their bodies." This rises to 78 percent by the time a girl reaches age seventeen.[7]

I am seriously troubled by this. I am the mother of two teenage girls, and I remember being a teenager who felt miserable in my skin. The accurate determination of what is appropriately thin for any girl or woman is relative to her frame. I am convinced as well that all individuals can achieve their own level of thinness, a healthy level. However, the level shown in the media is far from realistic or healthy. And, trust me, Hollywood knows it.

Think about the number of times you have read about a celebrity getting help for a dangerous eating disorder. Then eventually she writes a book about it and relaunches her career. I'm afraid for our daughters and for the baby girls being born as we speak. There needs to be a major shift. I have faced the fact that I will never be Twiggy or Kate Moss. We must keep drilling this into the minds of women and the impressionable young girls all around us. Stop trying to be someone else's best, and be your own!

Don't buy the lie of the world's deal. It offers nothing but drama and despair. Reject it. Call it a lie. And let's move on to the next chapter, where I'll offer you the best deal you could ever ask for.

4

God Offers You the Deal of a Lifetime

If You've Missed It in the Past, Don't Make the Same Mistake Again

I t's time to take a close look at the deal God offers you, and I admit it makes me nervous to write about something this critical to your success. Earlier I confessed what my deal used to be and all the struggles it produced. We talked about what your deal might be, based on what I hear regularly from clients and readers. But when it comes to God and what He offers us, I can't find big enough words to describe it all.

I know this for sure: God's deal is much greater than any of us can imagine. I keep learning new things about His faithfulness, and I'm blown away again and again by His goodness and grace. I also know that for entirely too long I missed what He was offering me. I always tried to make things happen on my own. I would make plans, work hard to implement them, and then fail—again and again. I was trying so hard to control things that I missed the importance of surrender. Sure, if you had asked me back then if I had yielded my whole life to God, I would have told you, "Of course!" But I know now that I was totally clueless. All my efforts to control kept leading to pain and disappointment. At one point I wondered if I had broken God's heart one time too many, mostly because I kept struggling with the same temptations and kept making the same mistakes.

Please Listen Closely...

But that was then. I have learned a lot since, and every day I continue to learn more about the true love of God. I've caught a glimpse of what God has in store for every one of us, and it is jaw dropping! God's deal for you and me is pure, perfect, and full of passion. It cannot be duplicated by any other offer, no matter what someone might promise. God's deal is nothing less than the one thing we all need and search for but fear we'll never find. God offers us love that is limitless. It's a love that is uninhibited and completely undeserved. And God gives it to us freely, knowing we can do nothing to earn it.

This is the real deal of our Dad, Abba Father. *What He wants more than anything is for us to grasp His true and perfect love!* Grasping His deal is the first baby step in learning how to walk through life hand in hand with the Savior.

You may be asking, "What's love got to do, got to do with it?"[1] when it comes to maintaining your weight and staying fit. I can hear some of you saying, "Chantel, I don't need a sermon. I just need to get into a bathing suit by summer." My response is that without first accepting God's deal, you'll put yourself at a disadvantage. You will hamper your ability to reach your highest goals and deepest longings in life. And believe it or not, that also includes finding the perfect swimsuit (an oxymoron, by the way). Without grasping God's perfect love, all of us will try to fix our lives on our own, and we'll fail once again. If experience teaches us anything, it's that we are limited and inconsistent, even when our plans are well intentioned.

The last thing I want to do is be a part of helping you obtain temporary success or, even worse, ultimate failure. So here is how you can stop this before it happens. First, face up to your shortcomings. Work hard at making a plan and setting goals, then determine to stay the course for the rest of your life. This is not an experiment or a short-term adventure. This is a new life!

Having said that, once you begin your new life, I can promise you there will be setbacks and temporary failures. So don't forget that occasionally falling short reminds us that we are imperfect and that we desperately need God's help. It keeps us needing Him. He wants us to have what is ultimately best for us, but He won't force it on us. Our free will is what enables us to love Him on the deepest levels humanly possible. But it also allows us to consume an entire bag of chips at one sitting.

God is interested in your fitness and overall health and well-being in ways you can't imagine. Before I gave birth to each of my children, I already loved them. I began to do things that contributed to their health long before they were born. And once they entered the world, the love kept growing. The love I have for my kids makes me care about anything that might cause them physical or emotional pain. Every scrape from a fall, fever in the night, and bump on the head still brings me to my knees. Not to mention the occasional worry that something more serious could be going on. As their mommy, I need reassurance that God is in control. So I ask Him to care for my children.

Now I want you to picture God, the perfect Father. Can you imagine how He feels when He watches us struggle with our bruised and battered hearts and bodies? How must He feel when He sees our physical suffering related to weight issues? According to Psalm 139:13–16, He is the One who created the frame that is carrying your body and mine!

HELPING ANOTHER PERSON GET IT

Recently my daughter Ashley went with me to Washington DC for a speaking engagement. We had a good laugh while she stood behind the merchandise table at the conference. Teenage boys came by from time to time and asked for her autograph. They were looking for a way to meet her, and it gave me a chance to talk to my teenager about the world of flirting. (At the time the awkward attention the boys paid my daughter was cute and gave us a good laugh. Not so much in the future, I'm sure.)

I planned an extra day for us to shop and sightsee. I wanted to take Ashley to Arlington National Cemetery to help her understand the ultimate act of patriotism. In this historic national cemetery, and with our country at war, I thought she should understand the real meaning of sacrifice.

If only it were that simple. I was aggravated by Ashley's casual attitude, marked by the constant questioning of exactly how many minutes we would be there. From the moment we stepped out of the rental car, she let me know this place that marks the ultimate sacrifice for freedom was of no interest to her. And in only a few minutes I was sobbing. The overwhelming emotion at first was mostly my trying to figure out where I had failed as a parent. Did I forget to teach Ashley all the words to "The Star Spangled Banner"? Should we have recited the Pledge of Allegiance more frequently?

Really, why was she acting more concerned about her fashion statement for the afternoon than about being an American? As we looked over the countless headstones of fallen soldiers, she continued to ask how long we were going to stay. At this point I informed her that I was contemplating spending the night there, just to prove we would leave when I was ready. I found myself echoing my mom's voice more loudly as I made an emotional speech at the eternal flame that burns at John F. Kennedy's grave. I went on and on, talking about mothers who lost their sons and describing the sacrifice of war heroes. As tears streamed down my face, I realized all we needed were bagpipes and a flag-folding ceremony to complete my American-pride experience.

Finally, when Ashley continued to show no emotion, I did something else my mom might have done. I called my husband, Keith. Mom for sure would have phoned Dad if she'd had a cell phone when I was a teenager. I said, "Do something with your daughter. She doesn't get it."

He said, "What do you expect, Chan? She's fourteen. It takes time. Trust me, you didn't get it either at fourteen."

So I let Ashley win, and we moved on. Our next stop was the Jefferson Memorial. I told her to chill out or we would never get to the shopping. My daughter is a cheerleader and an active girl, but when it comes to walking long distances—like more than a block—she acts like a ninety-year-old woman. I had to listen to her complaints during the entire ten-minute walk. I decided I wouldn't let her attitude steal any more of my "I'm proud to be an American" moments. I wanted to remind her that we do hold these truths to be self-evident, even if she was busy being self-absorbed.

Then it happened, the breakthrough I'd been hoping for. Ashley and I raced up the marble stairs and looked at the statue of Thomas Jefferson. As we stared up at the walls surrounding it, we took turns reading the words with awe. I vaguely remember studying the Declaration of Independence in American history class in high school, like around ten years ago, give or take another ten. However, there is a strong possibility I was more interested in the boy who sat behind me than I was in grasping the true meaning of this proclamation.

But on this cool, crisp fall day in Washington DC, I experienced a historic mother-daughter moment. Reciting the words with my child meant much more to me than I can say. They spoke of the need to uphold the belief in God as our Creator. And they reminded us of His provision and His desire to protect and preserve equality for all people.

Ashley said to me, "It seems most people have forgotten all this, and about God, doesn't it, Mommy?" I bowed my head in obvious agreement. Our society has strayed far from upholding these American ideals.

In the car afterward, driving back to our hotel, I talked to my firstborn about God's love and the protection we all need for our lives. I shared how God has fashioned us to need Him for everything. (Just saying the word *fashion* got her attention.) I also told her that without Him, we have no peace. He is the centerpiece to the puzzle of life. We know the Bible teaches these things, but history reminds us of the same things.

I believe our lives reveal this truth to us. We make our own decisions and choices, and often we see our choices lead us down dead ends, reminding us of how much we need God's love, direction, and help. Without His love and guidance, we soon fall apart.

STRENGTH BEYOND YOUR OWN

And that brings us back to the deal God is offering you. It's the perfect deal for every one of us, and it requires that we grab hold of two things.

But before we do, we must understand that God gives us freedom, which has the potential for different outcomes. Since we are free to run our own lives, we often try to do so for a time and end up in frustration and failure. The best outcome of the freedom God gives us occurs when we freely seek and accept His help. Ultimate freedom happens if we accept the plan and purpose God intends for our lives and allow Him to be in charge instead of us.

Choosing God-directed freedom also releases us from self-imposed bondage. For years I lived in bondage to my low self-esteem and out-of-control weight problem. Forget my compromised physical health, which was a given. My spiritual health was declining rapidly. I was sinking in self-hatred and had basically given up on God's desire to rescue me.

Eventually I had no strength left to rescue myself. In prior years I had mustered the energy necessary to try new diets. I could even feel okay for a few minutes by applying more lipstick. I could force a smile when yet another person insisted on saying, "You have such a pretty face." But that finally came to an end. One night I was done with all the false promises offered by quick fixes. That's when I was ready to accept God's deal. Maybe you are there too.

Two fundamental truths—think of them as two deal points—brought me back to God. Or perhaps the deal points introduced me to God in a way I had never known Him before. The first is that we must grasp the extent and power of God's love for us. The second is that it's futile to try to do life on our own. We will fail every time.

First things first: God loves you in a way that far exceeds even the strongest, most extravagant human love. God's love is pure and unpretentious. You will never be able to deserve or earn it. But if you choose to embrace God's love, it will heal you in every area where you hurt. God's love is so overwhelming that it's not easy to believe or to accept. Part of the difficulty arises from our lack of faith in God and His love, and part of it is our natural bent toward disobedience. All of us by nature are weak and flawed. Even when we learn what God wants for our lives, we tend to reject it in favor of our own desires and understanding.

Being overweight was my greatest life struggle. However, many people deal with sin they don't wear, so it's not as obvious. Even when it comes to an unhealthy obsession such as abusing food, you may never know it by the looks of their bodies. No matter what our issues are, we all are flawed, weak, and powerless over the things that control us. There is nothing we can do to impress God in order to convince Him that He should love us. He loves us already, far more than we can ever love ourselves. Even when I lost two hundred pounds, God didn't start loving me more. We can't get more of God's love by improving ourselves. We already have all of His love. The difference is that we don't know the benefit of His love until we grasp the way He loves us. Grasping the depth and extent of God's love for me gave me the will to succeed in weight loss, in fitness, and in changing my life. It gave me the desire to please God and to thank Him for my body, which is a gift.

God's love for you makes all the difference when you face up to the second deal point: trying to do life on our own is futile. None of us is smart enough, strong enough, disciplined enough, or righteous enough to live the life we dream of. But if you admit your inadequacies and imperfections and are humble enough to seek God's love and help, He will come through for you. With God, you gain the realistic hope that you can overcome your struggles, both small and gigantic. For me it began with attacking my weight problem and food issues. But I never would have succeeded without a complete reliance on God. If I had tried it under my own power, I would have found myself back in bondage and being overweight for the hundredth time.

Seriously consider both deal points. Gain an understanding of the way God loves you, and admit the futility of trying to do life on your own, without God. If you can grasp both points, the ultimate Deal Maker will work in your life in ways you never imagined possible.

How to Accept the Deal God Offers You

God's deal for you is powerful and necessary, but simple and straightforward. You can accept the freedom to love food and live well for a lifetime by making five decisions. These are the same five decisions I made years ago, the ones that made my own transformation stick! They also provide the path that can lead to your ultimate victory.

(Before you read any further, please take a moment to make sure it's a time when you can fully digest what I'm about to share. This means you should take a break from this book if you are trying to nurse a newborn, cook dinner, manage homework, or update your Facebook page. When you are able to devote some time to what I have to say, go to a quiet place where you can be alone and seriously consider the following.)

Decide if you are ready to be truthful with yourself and with God and to face the funk in your life. The funk includes all the things you never seem to gain victory over. Perhaps it's your weight, food addiction, or compulsive behavior. Only you really know what is constantly trying to steal your joy. Perhaps your life hasn't turned out the way you imagined it would. Do you realize that your old failures will blind you from seeing the love of God? If you are ready to stop struggling, believe today that Jesus came to save you from your sins, and you can now have victory over every stronghold or addiction in your life.

Pray and ask God to help you. And if you have already accepted Him as your Lord but can't seem to make it to the other side in a particular area, perhaps it's time to recommit your entire life to Him. This doesn't mean you have been living a lie; it means perhaps you've been holding something back. Romans 8:37 tells us we are "more than conquerors through him who loved us" (NIV). Therefore, the real question is, Are you truthfully willing to let God lead you into this battle, and will you choose to follow and be obedient, like a soldier? Even if this means doing some hard things that will challenge you...

If you are ready, start by recognizing that the love of God caused Him to send His Son to earth to die for your sin (see John 3:16). Salvation from your shortcomings and screwups is why Jesus showed up on the earth.

Next, if you acknowledge that you need His help and are ready to profess your belief in Him, *you'll need to repent and ask for forgiveness.* All your bad habits, hang-ups, sins, and failures can be forgotten today if you will cry out to Him and accept His forgiveness. No one is smart enough to run his or her own life, so by accepting God's love and forgiveness, you are surrendering to His control. This sets you free from your failed efforts to run your own life, and it plugs you into God's power to resist temptation.

Then, with complete honesty and the joy of realizing the meaning of God's forgiveness and redemption, *make a no-holds-barred commitment.* You are letting God take control, and as you do that, you are committing your full cooperation for the rest of your life. Don't expect a stress-free and temptation-free life. Changing your life is hard work. Remember, you are now marching in God's army!

Next, *you need to decide to seek knowledge.* Information gives you power to make solid decisions. This means you must take a deep, personal interest in how God has rigged you from the inside out, which includes learning about nutrition, how your body works, and how exercise contributes to health and well-being. This book will serve as a playbook for you to do this.

And last, to really see God's deal have a permanent effect on your life, you need insurance that your choices will stick. The deal you are going to receive is this: you can be free to love food and live well for a lifetime! And because it's a new life that lasts, you can't opt out of it. If you do, you will risk everything.

I know from experience that when people decide to change their lives, whether it's to get healthy, lose weight, or make another major change, they usually fail because they think they can manage it the old way. That's why you need the guarantee of knowing that *surrendering to the living God your life, your own strength, and your ability to change is a daily occurrence.* You have to lay down your desires whenever they get in the way of what God wants to do in your life. Remember, your personal desires and feelings, your sense of discouragement or frustration will always threaten to defeat you. Don't allow anything to block God's best for you. This life is going to reap health and utter freedom forever!

Today you can claim the deal God offers you. No, you won't lose all the excess weight you may be carrying. But you will be released from the burden of worrying if it's going to happen because now you aren't doing it alone. Not only does God's deal carry throughout your days on earth; it extends into eternity. I had to get to the end of my rope and abandon my own deal, which had brought nothing but failure and defeat. I also had to stop believing the world's deal, which convinced me I was worthless, lacking, and of no value. Will you do the same?

Remember, God's deal is always a win-win proposition. He wins your heart, and then you receive freedom on earth and an eternity with Him.

With these decisions made, you have surrendered to God, and He has promised His love and power to you. Now every God-given pleasure, including a brownie, is for your enjoyment! Let the power of God's deal take over. You will find the thrill and strength of loving food and living well, starting today and lasting for a lifetime.

PART 2

Start Your
New Life Today

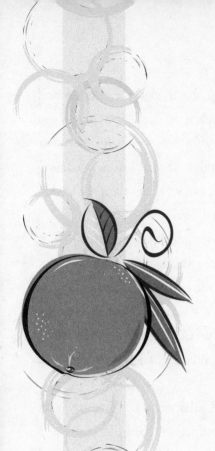

5

Which Deal Will You Take?

The Next Step Is Choosing the Life You Want

*I*f you have ever bought a car, a set of used dishes at a garage sale, or a new washer, you know about negotiating. It's impossible to carry out a transaction or finalize a contract without coming to terms. When you negotiate terms, it means you have decided to act, and you're putting something behind it.

Car shopping is one of life's greatest tortures. It's like getting a root canal—necessary, painful, and expensive! I'm convinced that a lot of the torment in car buying comes from all the decisions you have to make simultaneously: choosing the model, the features and options, and don't forget the color. It's too much at one time. It all makes you want to hyperventilate. But a car is necessary for most of us. So every few years I suck it up and go to the showrooms and do the hard work of coming to terms with a salesperson. It's never painless, but it's better than not having transportation. And every time I have survived.

Think back to the last time you spent a lot of money on something. It might have been a car, a major appliance, a remodeling project, or landscaping. The dreaded negotiation process starts with window-shopping. When you need to replace a car, the shopping begins by checking out the vehicles you see on the road. Next, you might read what *Consumer Reports* has to say. Thankfully, they've already done the legwork on safety and value. Then you pop by a dealership just to take a peek.

That's when you're exposed, vulnerable. A salesperson walks up and asks your name. You have to make a formal introduction. (Feel like you're at a junior high dance?) In about three minutes a "courtship" has begun, pressed by one of the ten men who rushed out to greet you in the dealer's parking lot. Within fifteen minutes you're on a test drive and already asking yourself, *Am I in love?* No need to worry if the salesman is going to call after the first date. He probably took down your number before he got your name.

You notice he makes no serious effort during the road test to discuss the price of this little beauty. He seems to care only about how you are feeling. "How's the driving position? Do you find the seats comfortable? That GPS system is almost as good as a police escort. I'll bet your sound system at home doesn't make Céline Dion sound this good. And did you check the legroom in back? Your kids will finally stop complaining that they're cramped. Plus, they'll be engrossed in the movie you play on the DVD, shown on a flatscreen for backseat passengers."

You're thinking, *Wow, this guy really understands the challenges facing a modern woman.*

The salesperson wants you to bond with the car. "How does she feel when you step on the gas?" he asks. *Hmm,* you think, *that's sweet. This shiny new vehicle is a she.* You can picture a long and enduring friendship with her. She will be a new girlfriend. You can hang out with her in the carpool line. You can feel comfortable enough with her to yell when someone cuts you off in traffic. She will let you order the chocolate milkshake and cheeseburger in the drive-through and say nothing about it. You haven't even pulled back into the dealer's lot, and already you love her.

All you can think about is how good she smells, clean and new. Your old car has a bad odor, although you admit some fault for leaving a bottle of milk under the seat.

The test drive is over, and this flashy new model has passed the test. As you walk into the showroom, the aroma of buttery popcorn is overwhelming. Your love for this new car has sharpened all your senses. Your love has officially turned to lust. *It's all good,* you begin to think.

In a trancelike state, you are led to an office where reality hits. You face the fact that feeling this good isn't free. Sitting down in the finance office, you gaze out the window at your new best friend. She is waiting for you, wanting to hang out. You find that you want this relationship to work, so you ask the crucial question: "What's the best price you can give me"?

Sure, I have asked it too. So has everyone else who has taken a car for a test drive. So much for your tricky negotiating technique. Did you think your bold question would somehow give you the upper hand and produce a bottom-line price more in your favor?

Lucky for you, you happened to stop by on the day when the dealer is having a "once in a millennium, Saturday after sunset, hurricane–Super

Bowl closeout sale special." So you strike a deal. You come to terms. She is coming home to live with you.

THE REALITY OF COMING TO TERMS

When you finally close the deal, three things happen. First, you decide this car is the one you really want. (You made that decision after carefully considering the cost, right?) Second, you hand over some money as a down payment, which says you are fully committed to keeping your end of the bargain. Finally, as you are handed the car keys, you are free to leave with your new purchase. For a brief second your stomach may turn. You hope you made the right choice. But as you drive away, it doesn't matter all that much. She is shiny and smells good, and all your friends will think she's cool.

A few weeks later reality finally hits. The payment book arrives. Throwing it in the trash is not an option. You have to make payments on the loan every month. It's going to be painful to hand over that much money every thirty days. But the choice was yours, you negotiated the price, and you accepted ownership.

Buying a car is just one of many areas in which we do background research, make a decision, and come to terms with the decision we made. Deal making comes in many forms every day for all of us. I can't think of anyone who illustrates this better than my new friend Margie.

Margie wasn't shopping for a new car, but she did set out to find a new life. And she came to terms out of utter desperation. (I know the feeling well.) I met Margie through one of my sisters-in-law. I was told prior to meeting her that she had an amazing story to share. When we first met, I'll admit I was caught off guard. She grabbed me, hugged me, and proceeded to sob. I actually thought this woman might not let go of me. I was intensely touched by her emotion; I just wasn't sure why there was so much of it.

As you might guess, Margie had me at *hello.* She held a copy of my first book, *Never Say Diet,* in one hand and a black Sharpie in the other. She began wiping away tears as she asked me to sign the book. She said meeting me was a celebration of her fiftieth birthday. I was wondering why she hadn't chosen a day at the spa or maybe a new pair of shoes. But here she was, asking for my autograph. I joyfully obliged, and as I opened the book, I was overwhelmed with emotion. I saw that Margie had underlined sentence after sentence. She had even written notes in the margins.

Coming to terms and closing the deal starts with a "brain change." That is when you decide you want a new life and you will allow nothing to stop you. You promise to tell yourself the truth, you ditch all your old excuses, and you pursue your new life without compromise or conditions. The date Margie began her Brain Change was marked in bold letters. She had also taped photographs inside, showing her before she came to terms and then her now enjoying her new life. The difference was distinct.

I also noticed that the binding of the book was beginning to look like an old, used-up novel from a public library or a secondhand store. I was humbled to think that the words I had written meant so much to this stranger.

Margie took me back to the main event in her life: New Year's Eve, 2007. That was the night her life shattered and her marriage fell apart. Instead of blowing horns, throwing confetti, and singing "Auld Lang Syne" to welcome in the new year, she had nothing and no one to welcome. Her husband and business partner of more than thirty years chose New Year's Eve to tell her he was leaving. He also disclosed his plans to reunite with an old high school flame who lived out of state.

Margie had known that she and her husband had communication issues, but divorce had never been on the table. Suddenly, the decision was being made without her. Margie's husband packed up and took off to rekindle a romance of days gone by. She was left packing as well. But hers was emotional baggage. She started to carry around an unbearable load of pain. Margie was desperate for just one day to pass without feeling rejected and alone.

This woman poured out her heart to me, describing the feeling of being abandoned, mourning a broken home, and coping with her shattered heart. Hearing her story broke my heart as well. For the first time in decades, Margie was running the business and living as a single woman. Her life had been turned upside down, and she still didn't have an explanation.

On top of all the pain and confusion, she was seriously overweight and apprehensive about her fiftieth birthday, which was quickly approaching. With her life in shambles, feeling betrayed, Margie did the only thing she could: she cried out to God. Then my book showed up. It was God's perfect timing for her: His message of grace packaged with a practical plan for action. He had heard her cry. I had obeyed God by writing about the deliverance from my own lifelong struggle. I wrote the book because He had shown me there were countless Margies in this world.

Whether you are starting your first diet and fitness program, your fifth, or your fiftieth, you have to make your own deal. As Margie told me her story, she explained what her deal was and the new deal she came to terms with. She could choose to stay on the road she had traveled for years and undoubtedly end up a bitter person, or she could seriously consider the deal God was offering her. Margie chose her Creator. She knew He had been whispering her name for quite some time, and after she read my story of His faithfulness, she couldn't deny it. Margie was tired; God wanted to give her rest. She was a victim of fear and anger; He wanted to comfort and protect her. She chose to welcome the gifts He offered.

You have the same choice. You can stay on the road you've been traveling and keep the life you already have. Or you can come to terms with God and accept the deal He is offering you.

The night I met Margie, she was free, fit, fifty pounds lighter, and a stunning fifty-year-old woman. But, most important, she was a woman who knew she had been rescued. This gave her a passion for sharing her story of deliverance and the faithfulness of God.

As she shared her joy, I noticed that she never once expressed a wish for her life to be different. She didn't say, "Oh to be twenty years younger," or "I just want to be a little skinnier." This night she could only describe the power of love, forgiveness, and living well. She was overflowing with joy.

You may identify more with Margie's story than mine, but the message remains the same. We both finally chose to stop running the show when we decided to change our lives. We came to terms, closed the deal, and got to work. That work involved making the hard decisions to own up to our deficiencies by being truthful about our flaws, to commit to a "no excuses, no matter what" mentality, and to learn how to love food properly. By seeking a surrendered heart every day, neither one of us will ever be the same. The unconditional love of God first rescued us. Then His teaching us how to let Him control our lives became the glue that made the deal and now holds it together.

It's Time to Close the Deal

You need to become familiar with the deal points. This is the list of what you are giving and getting as a result of making the deal. Then you must commit to fulfill all the terms of the deal. Remember, you are making the deal of a lifetime to love food and live well—a deal that will deliver the new life you desire.

To make your new deal stick, it's important that you grasp the intensity and bigness of God's love for you. In this deal, you are receiving His pure love. It is limitless. In return, you are giving up old hurt, bitterness, and disappointment. To lay hold of your new life, you have to let go of your old life. If you can't do this yet, you're not ready to make the deal. You also need to realize and acknowledge that God's limitless love is a gift you don't deserve and can't earn. It is a gift, and all you can do is accept it. This means you will stop trying to be good enough to earn God's love. You can never do enough good things, say enough good things, live a good-enough life, or even lose enough weight to deserve it.

You can't do life well enough alone. You need God's help.

This is the meaning of surrender, which we talked about in chapter 4. It is simple, but it is also the hardest thing you will ever do. You give up the right to be in charge. From now on, you give over control of your life to God. In giving up the frustration of trying to rule your own life, you receive the gift of freedom. This deal makes the difference between trying again and succeeding and trying again and failing again to lose weight, get healthy, and stay fit for the rest of your life. Making the deal—surrendering to God and accepting the deal He offers—is the solution to food addiction, yo-yo dieting, a negative self-image, struggles with body image, and every other area of bondage.

If you are ready, let's get started by defining your expectations.

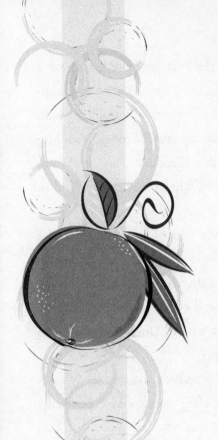

6

Define Your Expectations Now!

What Do You Really Want Out of Life?

*L*et's say it's possible to get what you really want. What would you be willing to pay? And, closer to home, what would you be willing to give up?

The first step is to define what you really want, deep down, for your life. What does it mean to live well? Do you need a Ferrari life, or can you live well with less than that?

I've never negotiated the purchase of a Ferrari.

Sure, I can imagine myself cruising down the Fort Lauderdale strip on a cloudless day at the wheel of a little cherry red number with a spotless, non-crayoned, tan leather interior. The wind is blowing gently through my hair. I begin to serenade the entire city, belting out my favorite songs. It's a new pastime I've created in my mind: convertible karaoke! Okay, sorry, I'm back. I really do know the difference between fantasy and reality. And so do you.

The truth is that a sports car would never fit my lifestyle. It won't seat four kids, let alone their nine friends who seem to always tag along. Actually, just paying the taxes on a Ferrari would be a stretch. Then there would be the monthly payment. According to my husband—the "budget bully" at our house—our mortgage must always win. I accept it. My fantasy has no chance of becoming reality, at least not anytime soon.

So what things make up a great life that are realistic and doable? What is within reach that will produce a life far exceeding what you've experienced until now?

Do You Have the Right Dream?

It's good to dream, since we all want to improve ourselves and get the most out of life. Without dreams we wouldn't be stirred to do the things that will move us from where we are to where we want to be. So let's look at dreams.

When I weighed over 350 pounds and made my "no going back" commitment to losing weight and getting healthy, I didn't set out to wear a size 2 or to weigh 125 pounds. My frame is not designed for either of these goals. Even though I was dead serious about achieving and maintaining a natural, healthy weight, I knew my commitment had to be realistic. For instance, I didn't make a crazy commitment to give up sugar for the rest of my life. That would have meant no birthday cake—ever! Come on! I'm the queen of celebration. I love nothing more than throwing a party.

I'm also a wife and a mom with a career and family responsibilities. In other words, I'm a real person just like you. I could never eat an all-organic diet and shop at four grocery stores just to find everything I need at affordable prices so I can follow an unrealistic regimen. And committing to six hours of exercise a day in order to achieve crazy goals makes no sense either. With my genetics, body type, and available time, the bottom line is that my food and fitness program has to fit into a regular life.

So here's lesson one: when you dream about the life you want, dream in the real world. Many people are frazzled by trying to accomplish something they can't possibly attain. For months the news has been full of stories about the housing market and the rise in foreclosures. An astounding number of people signed papers for mortgages they couldn't pay. Likewise, too many of us believe we can achieve a fantasy. Lots of people suffer because of repossessed dreams and goals. They wanted a better life, but they set out to achieve a life that wasn't feasible.

I support dreaming big—how else can we challenge ourselves to be the absolute best we can be? If you have tried and failed to get fit and lose weight, don't accept the guilt of believing your yo-yo dieting is because you're a failure or a quitter. More likely you committed to the wrong dreams and goals. In a sense you failed before you even started. If you have trouble accepting this, then stop right now and think about your frustrated goals and the things you've given up on. Were they actually realistic and maintainable?

To bring about lasting changes in our lives, we need to accept the deal God is offering. We've seen before that our own deal was destined to fail. We have all suffered the fallout of giving it our best shot and failing anyway. So let's reorient our dreams to coincide with God's deal. God-given dreams are always attainable. Stop and reread the last sentence. I'm not saying they are small—they usually are dreams that stretch us beyond anything we thought possible. But they are within reach, and that's the big difference.

This is something that's difficult for me to admit, and I mention it only because I believe it will help you. There was a time after I lost the two hundred pounds when I struggled to understand the limits of my body. During those months I battled obsessive thoughts. Bear in mind that I had already lost the equivalent of more than an entire person! But I couldn't relax and enjoy the achievement of this dream.

I would regularly ask my husband, "Baby, do I need to lose more weight?" When I exercised, I couldn't stop wondering if one more squat or lunge would fix my problem areas, so I'd add more time to my already lengthy workouts. I had achieved amazing weight loss, and I had created an entire program that delivered sustainable weight loss and fitness, but none of it seemed to satisfy me at that time even though this was a couple of years after my weight had reached a set point, and I had sustained that weight. I was eating clean and sticking to an intense daily exercise program. But I couldn't accept where I was because I wasn't yet perfect.

After continued study I realized that all my extra effort didn't change reality. I had made remarkable changes in my life, but the perfect body I thought I needed was out of reach. I had to seriously let go. If I didn't surrender this to God, I knew I would risk total insanity. Honestly, I had reached a point that was scaring me.

This was not an easy decision. I had nurtured these dreams for years, and I had worked hard. Trust me, it wasn't easy to abandon my dreams of long, thin, shapely legs, but it was necessary. Defining real expectations has the power to set us free and show us that lifelong success can be attained and maintained.

So as you decide what life you seek, dream big but be realistic. You will still achieve far more than you ever have before and more than you ever dreamed was possible.

THE PERFECT DOWN PAYMENT

In the following chapters we will learn to love food while taking away its power over us. No longer will food defeat you, and no longer will your fear of food and attitudes about food sabotage your fitness and weight-loss success. Before we're finished, you will be free to eat food with passion and gusto.

However, the first step in this process is to come to terms with food. It requires taking a hard look, being honest with yourself, and being willing to pay the price. We will start with a fast, an ancient practice that is well known in religious circles. I don't mean *fast* in terms of quickness or a rush. Instead, this *fast* is a noun.

There are two ways to look at fasting, according to the dictionary. Fasting is abstaining from food for religious reasons or as a means of protest. I want you to consider both meanings. Many religions, from Christianity to Islam, observe seasons of corporate fasting. When you begin to choose your own deal of a lifetime with God, fasting is the perfect down payment. It says you are willing to pay the price, to sacrifice your wants, and go the distance. A fast can signify your intense desire to be closer to God. As you give up the will to eat for a short time, you give God the opportunity to satisfy your needs.

At the same time, you can protest the bondage you have felt to constantly trying to fulfill all your wants on your own. Many develop the habit of satisfying physical, spiritual, and emotional appetites by reaching for food. I promise that fasting will give you freedom from this.

When you are ready to embark on this deal, go for it. With fasting, you don't ease into it. It's a sudden thing, and it's simple. For twenty-four hours—from waking one morning to waking the next—drink only water and give up all food.

Many studies have shown the value of fasting. One major benefit is the clarity of thinking it delivers. As food leaves your system without replenishment, your brain shifts to survival mode. You don't enjoy the benefit of that clearer brain function when you keep feeding your appetites. But as this natural instinct powers up during a fasting period, your thinking becomes unclouded. Suddenly you find surprising solutions to life's challenges.

How many times have we heard of people who survived horrific circumstances by doing unthinkable things in order to stay alive? I have read of self-amputation, getting nourishment from a rat, and many other crazy scenarios. By the way, there is almost always a scarcity of food in these cases. Of course, this will not be quite the same for you, because your fast will last for only one day and one night. However, a day without eating can feel like a lifetime.

To get the greatest benefit from your one-day fast, add prayer. Ask God to help you live better. Talk to Him as your friend. Seek His help as you hand over your food struggles, low self-esteem, and anything else that keeps defeating you. The next day you will awake feeling revived. This fast will be a substantial symbol that you have come to terms with accepting God's deal.

In the next few chapters, I will give you a better picture of everything we eat and how to plan your food choices. In the meantime, start preparing to reestablish your relationship with food. How you relate to food is a revealing, eye-opening, life-changing picture of your fixations and loss of control.

Gaining the ability to make decisions regarding eating is a big step in personal power. Food choices are driven by need, which makes the power that food holds over us intense. But, likewise, when we gain control over our relationship with food, we gain an intense increase in personal strength. When you surrender your struggle with food to God and rely on His help to give you the control you seek, you experience freedom.

What's next? Will your food cravings disappear? (I wish.) Will all temptations cease? (Not likely.) Food is here to stay. Since we can't survive without it, food can be more difficult to set aside than a drug. Food is essential, it's legal, and in our society it's always within reach. Food seems so innocent, so harmless, that it's easy to maintain a flawed perspective. Food is not evil; it's necessary and God-given. It's just our relationship with food that becomes skewed. The key to getting healthy in your eating is to love food properly, which is exactly what I will teach you how to do.

Don't Fall for Their Tricks

Remember my friend Margie from chapter 5? (She's the woman whose life fell apart when she turned fifty and her husband decided to dissolve their marriage.) As she began to chart a new course for her life, she had to be truthful. That included giving up all her old excuses and moving forward with a promise to never lie to herself again. This is the first decision in the Brain Change process. (For more on the Brain Change, see my book *Never Say Diet*.[1]) Margie had to face the reality that even though she was brokenhearted over her husband leaving her, she was also overweight. Margie knew it would take a long time for her heart to heal and trust again, but she could tackle fitness and weight loss immediately.

As she began to shift her mind, she made the commitment that food would no longer be her source of comfort, her source of entertainment, or her best friend. Starting that day, food would be nothing more than a source of fuel and energy. As you launch a life change, food cannot be your means to immediate happiness or the source of emotional gratification. For now, you have to make food boring. Diets that pitch a plan for you to eat your favorite food and lose weight at the same time are a joke. When solving a problem, you can't continue to feed the root of your problem.

I'm not making light of your struggle with food. I know firsthand that this is no laughing matter. Lots of weight-loss plans promise that you can change your life without making major changes. They sell customers on the idea that change is easy, that it requires little sacrifice, and that you can have a new life by basically continuing all your old habits, which is what led to your problems. Rational people know that you don't change anything when you continue old habits. It's dishonest to pretend that you can, and, remember, we have promised to tell ourselves the truth.

Your favorite foods became your favorites because you loved them too much and too often. And your love of those foods has shown up unfavorably on your body. That's what you want to change, right? So the first step is a difficult but necessary one. You need to let go of your favorite foods for a while. Margie's fifty-pound weight loss and my weight loss were accomplished because we accepted a truth. Think about this and then repeat it to yourself: Food has never, ever solved any of my problems. Recite this slowly. Then repeat it so it will sink in.

When we eat whatever we want, whenever we want it, and without limitation, we get the very thing we are trying to get rid of. Eating stole our health and our fitness and our body. Eating delivered misery, not the life we long for. This is why Margie related to my story despite the differences in our circumstances. We were both done with feeling miserable and trapped. Can you relate? Both of us also had to learn about solid nutrition—food that delivers maximum energy—and how to get reacquainted with food as fuel and not as an intimate friend. By learning about food, the truth begins to stick and our eating habits change.

Beginning with chapter 7, we will become more informed about the properties of food. By taking in this information, your meals will match your new mind-set. The desire to feel better, look better, and live better will take over. Carbohydrates, protein, fats, french fries, and even brownies have a real place in the food pyramid. That truth can become part of your reality after you do the hard work of breaking your unhealthy love affair with food.

Before we tackle nutrition, though, I want to help you assess what is realistic for you to achieve according to your body structure. How much weight can you realistically lose? What weight can you maintain? More important, what weight is healthy and natural for your height and body type? This will be one marker for you of living well. We'll begin with your frame.

How to Love Your Own Body

If your goal is to compete next year in the Mrs. America Pageant, you may want to reconsider. I can save you the entry fee and the cost of an overpriced evening gown. Unless your proportions fall within a tiny fraction of a percentage of women aged thirty and over, you don't stand a chance. So let's get real and talk about the majority of women who have children, work for a living, and want to lose weight in a sustainable way. You might be shaped like a pear and dream of turning into an hourglass. Think about this: you probably have a greater chance of growing taller and switching your eye color.

This is where goals and dreams meet reality. You can change your life in dramatic ways, ways that exceed what you once thought was possible and ways that will impress your friends, your family, and yourself. But it starts with an honest self-evaluation, which is a key to making a total plan for lasting fitness and overall wellness. If you want to love food and live well, let's start by getting real.

It's important to define your level of contentment with your body as it is. Then determine how you can improve this level of contentment. Understanding your level of contentment or dissatisfaction will help you start to think differently. It's not "I'm always on a diet" or "It seems I always need to lose ten pounds." Now you'll think, "I respect my body, I work hard, I practice self-control, and I have found contentment with my frame. It's the body God designed for me."

I meet too many women who seem to believe that God made a mistake when He created them. If you listen to them talk about their bodies, you'll conclude that God was distracted when He accidentally gave them small breasts, overlarge breasts, or too wide a bottom, or when He made them short-waisted, too tall, too thin, or too whatever. It's time to get over that type of thinking. Read Psalm 139:13–16. These are my life's verses. They have given me peace more times that I can recall. God created you and me and everyone else before we were born. He "knit" us in our mothers' wombs. He took great care in making us exactly who we are. He didn't make a mistake with you, me, or anyone else.

If you can't accept your frame, your basic body type, and your general looks, then you will never be able to live well. Living well includes peace of mind, self-acceptance, and the ability to trust God, believing that He loves you, cares for you, and is on your side. In contrast to living well, I see too many women who believe that dropping to a size 6 will solve all their problems. These are the women who continue to feel frazzled, like they are in prison, even after they lose significant weight.

Listen, we have all been guilty of allowing others' expectations to determine how we feel about ourselves. Why give someone else the power to dictate a magical number that you feel you have to reach on the scale? I have met women who allowed another person to give them self-esteem or to rob them of it. Don't give anyone but God power over you. People will judge you based on physical beauty, weight, or shape. Sometimes it's a husband, boyfriend, or parent. Listen closely: your worth and true beauty can't be calculated by another person. I don't care what *Cosmo* says that contradicts what I'm telling you; it's a ploy to steal your money and sell magazines. Why do you think women's magazines keep telling you that you're not good enough? They can stay in business only as long as they make you believe you need their help and advice.

This is reality: all clocks keep ticking, life produces change, and outer beauty fades. You can't be eighteen forever. You can't have children and still look like a gymnast. Your skin will not be as smooth as it was when you were twenty. It might be hard to face these facts, but there is a reward in getting real about your appearance. The reward is this: you finally believe you were divinely created by a perfect God. Now don't misinterpret me as saying that it's all right to be fat and sassy as long as you love God. I don't believe anyone can be happy at an unhealthy weight. Plain and simple, it's not true.

The key to fitness, a healthy weight, and accepting your body is to determine the body type that God gave you and then go from there. So, first, we're going to define your body type. Body type is something you can't change; it is basically as fixed as your height. It is based on your bone structure and frame. But those who are carrying a significant amount of extra weight may have their body type misdiagnosed. It's not true that everyone who is overweight is big-boned. I had been told this my entire life, and I relied on that excuse for far too long. The truth is, I'm pretty much average. I am a five-foot-nine-inch-tall woman who could never be a runway model. Even if I chose to embark on a water-only, yearlong fast, I still would never gain another three inches in height. I am, however, proportionate after losing two hundred pounds, and I am an hourglass by definition. I have maintained a healthy body weight and a lower-than-average body fat percentage, and I wear a size 8 in most jeans.

This is me, not you. I don't tell you my story to brag, but simply to give you an example of a weight-loss success that got me to a healthy, sustainable weight. I share my story also to help you understand what it takes to be content and at peace with your body. Be yourself. Stop trying to be someone else.

DISCOVER YOUR BODY TYPE

There are four shapes of women's bodies. As I describe them, determine which one you match most closely. You may find it handy to have a measuring tape, paper, pencil, and calculator close by. They are banana, apple, pear, and hourglass. The shapes are defined according to chest, waist, and hip ratios.

Your body shape depends on your skeletal structure and the distribution of fat and muscle. To discover your body type, measure your bust around the fullest part of the breast. Measure your waist at the smallest part of your abdomen. Your hip measurement is the largest circumference around your buttocks. A woman's body dimension is determined by these three numbers. The ratio of chest measurement to waist measurement determines your body type. The legendary sex kitten with a thirty-six-inch chest, twenty-four-inch waist, and thirty-six-inch hips—a fantasy made popular in early James Bond movies and the overheated imaginations of pimply-faced teenage boys—is rarely seen in the real world. However, if you are such a woman, the ratio is 3:2:3, and the waist measurement is 66 percent the size of chest and hips. Those proportions exceed even the official definition of an hourglass shape. This is yet another example of the Barbie myth that has made so many women hate their bodies. Here are the four body-type ratios in greater detail.

The Banana

The waist circumference is at least 75 percent of the chest or hips, which makes the waist appear to be a similar size to the chest. Body fat tends to be distributed more around the waist. Many competitive athletes have this body type.

The Apple

The waist is at most 75 percent of the chest circumference, and the chest is at least 110 percent of the hip circumference. Body fat will be distributed first in the arms, shoulders, chest, and upper abdomen. As more fat accumulates, the lower abdomen also becomes enlarged. The apple body type carries fat in the legs and the buttocks last.

The Pear

The waist is at least 75 percent of the chest circumference, and the hip circumference is at least 110 percent of the chest circumference. The distribution of fat varies. Fat tends to be distributed first in the buttocks, hips, and thighs. As body fat increases, it eventually distributes itself into the waist and upper abdomen. However, this body type tends to accumulate saddlebags the quickest. This term is thought of as a disproportionate amount of fat on the sides of the thighs. The chest and arms are the last places to carry fat for a pear-shaped body.

The Hourglass

The waist circumference is 75 percent of the chest or hips, which are virtually the same size. Body fat tends to distribute evenly around the upper and lower body. This body distributes fat to enlarge arms, breasts, hips, and rear before any other part. The waist and upper abdomen are the last to store excess fat.

An interesting study carried out in 2005 by researchers at the University of North Carolina found that of six thousand women participants, 46 percent were banana, slightly more than 20 percent were pear, 14 percent were apple, and only 8 percent were hourglass.[2] As you assess your body type, recognize that any structure can occur in any range of proportions. In other words, no matter how overweight you are today, you can still determine your body type.

DETERMINE YOUR BODY FAT

A woman's ideal weight is often misunderstood and miscalculated, and body composition is the key factor behind this misunderstanding and miscalculation. Two people can weigh exactly the same but look entirely different. Our bodies are made up of fat, muscle, bone, and water. The variance in percentages between these four elements is what gives you your shape and determines how you look. It also explains why looking at a chart to determine your ideal body weight can lead to an unrealistic goal.

Remember, you are creating a picture in your mind of what living well looks like for you, not just for this year, but for the rest of your life. The best program for this is one where you maintain a healthy body-fat percentage. When you lose weight properly and do regular cardiovascular exercise and strength training, your lean muscle increases while body fat decreases.

There are several ways to determine body fat. Deciding which one to use is based on the resources you have available. The most accurate measurement is done hydrostatically, immersing you in water, but it can be expensive and difficult to find a facility to do this. Next, there are skin-fold measurements, which should be taken by a trained professional. The technician uses calipers to pinch several spots on your body and then by means of a formula determines your level of body fat. This method is the most accessible and is becoming more accurate with increased technological advances. Because body fat can be calculated by electromagnetic currents sent through your body, there are scales for sale that calculate body fat when you stand on them. They are way cool!

No matter how you decide to get an accurate idea of your best body goal, keep track regularly of your body-fat ratio, your measurements, weight, and body composition as a reference. This will aid you in keeping on track. Don't assume you are big-boned just because you are overweight, and don't set a goal of achieving an hourglass figure if you have a pear, an apple, or a banana shape because of your bone structure. Also, don't forget your frame is unique. Whether your frame matches your idea of perfection is irrelevant. Perfection is a perception, and God made you who you are.

PART 3

When It Comes to Food, Here Is the What and When

It's Time to Get a Clue About Calories

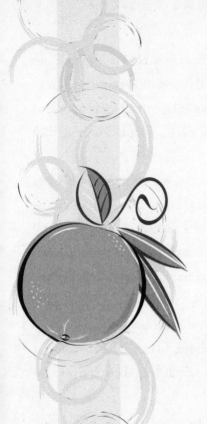

Find Out Which Foods Deliver the Biggest Benefits

W hen it comes to counting calories, most of us don't have a clue. At least that's what the International Food Information Council Foundation is reporting. According to one of the most dramatic findings in recent years, "nine out of 10 Americans are unable to accurately estimate the number of calories they should eat in an average day."[1] Meanwhile, *The American Journal of Preventative Medicine* reports that dietary information presented on food labels may be "well beyond" an individual's ability to understand, especially those with lower math skills.[2] Wow! While the government requires that detailed information be provided on every food label, most people can't understand it. That is assuming they even bother to glance at it.

If so many of us are unaware of the caloric content of the food we're eating, what does it mean for our health and fitness? For starters, I'm convinced that if we could read and quickly comprehend a food label, weight control would be much less of an issue. It's sad that 66.3 percent of Americans over the age of twenty are overweight.[3] Until a few years ago, I was one of the clueless 90 percent of the population. I thought the two-cookie serving recommendation on the Oreo package was only intended for small children. I also fit right into the data regarding obesity cited above. In fact, back then, about the only thing I fit into easily was the depressing statistics about the population of fat people in America.

Hallelujah, I finally woke up! Making the transition to living well, losing weight, and keeping it off became easier when I started to gain knowledge about calories. As I got a clue about the calories contained in different foods, especially in relation to their nutritional content, I recognized the power of food for the first time. Don't worry. I'm still going to show you how to love food. However, respect is a forerunner to loving anything really well. Respect is the utmost display of our ultimate intentions: to love everything that God gives us more fully. Because food fuels our bodies and because eating clean is essential, not just to weight loss, but also to energy, strength, endurance, and health, we need to learn how to respect food in a new way.

Respecting food has a lot to do with respecting yourself. Again, love and respect go hand in hand. When I was overweight, I couldn't have loved myself very much. I was regularly eating enough cookies to keep both the

Pillsbury Doughboy and the Keebler elves up all night baking. We all struggle with food, and educating ourselves about calories and nutrition is the first step in breaking the power that food has over us while getting the maximum benefit from food.

Here is a dose of reality. Think about a person whom you want to love and appreciate more. Now ask yourself if you respect this person for who he or she is. If you find that your level of respect is low, here is a way to elevate it.

Giving respect becomes more natural as you recognize how the other person operates. You begin to identify the benefits of that person's natural strengths and abilities. Consider your spouse, as just one example. Recall how you invested time in finding out the important things before your wedding. I knew my husband, Keith, cared deeply about managing his money. He was the only guy I had ever met who, at age sixteen, was diligent about paying bills. I can remember this boy cashing his paycheck from Service Merchandise and handing his parents the money for his long-distance phone charges before they even asked. (The calls were all to me, by the way.) He paid his bills before he would consider spending a dime on a pack of gum.

Trust me, I was annoyed at times by his sense of responsibility. Sometimes his lack of funds caused us to miss a date for dinner and a movie. Yet many times throughout the years of our marriage, I have thanked God that my husband is wired like this. If it weren't for him, I would probably have resorted to selling my blood for a new pair of shoes many times over. So instead, because I really like shoes, hate needles, and love my husband, I choose to discuss money and budgeting when he asks. (At least, I'm diligently working on it!)

Here's another example that's closely related to fuel, energy, and power. If, like me, you really enjoy getting around in a car, you are probably aware of a few automotive operating essentials. One, your car needs gas to go. Two, the engine must be serviced regularly. You can't enjoy your love for driving unless you also respect your car enough to take care of it. So respect yourself and your body enough to fuel it properly and to care for it.

How to Respect Food

Like your car, which requires the right fuel to perform at its best, your body needs the right food for maximum power. Because food is essential to your health, it is to be respected. You can choose to abuse food or to appreciate it and get the most from it.

To respect food, you must know what it's made of. The energy contained in food is measured by calories. In this chapter you will learn how calories function. By the way, a calorie by definition is the amount of heat needed to raise the temperature of a liter of water one degree. As it pertains to food, calories measure the energy in the food and liquids you consume. Everything we do is fueled by energy that comes from the caloric value of food and drink. Having the strength to live to the max, as well as to manage our weight, involves understanding how calories work.

It still amazes me when people say they are planning to lose weight without paying attention to calories. This is like saying, "I really want to have a baby. I just refuse to deal with dirty diapers and sleepless nights." Successfully losing weight for a lifetime won't happen without facing the reality of what you eat and how much you eat and learning what the food you eat does to your body. You must accept some inherent truths and respect them.

How to Get More Power

Because all food contains calories, all food supplies energy to your body. Think about it like this: a piece of chocolate contains much more energy than a piece of lettuce. Your body knows how to use what it needs, so when you consume more energy than is needed, your body stores the reserve to use later on. Storing up an energy reserve translates into weight gain, which explains why the quantity and timing of what you eat are the most important factors in successful weight maintenance. If you eat nothing but three chocolate bars a day, you won't become overweight. You will move around enough in one day to burn that many calories. However, try eating three chocolate bars every hour. Your weight will shoot up before you blink an eye. In contrast, you could eat nothing but a head of lettuce every fifteen minutes all day long, and you'd be trim forever. A calorie is the same amount of energy whether it comes from eating a carbohydrate, a protein, or a fat.

It is important to eat a proper balance of carbs, proteins, and fats because all three forms of nutrition serve different functions in your body. Consuming too many calories from one source before your body uses them will overload the system. Understanding the way carbs, protein, and fat work is essential for weight loss and maintenance, and we'll look at them in more detail later.

In the following chapters, I'll explain food, calories, and how they work in your body in a way that makes an often boring topic fun and informative. As you learn to love food and live well, you can laugh at the same time.

FALL IN LOVE WITH THE BEST CALORIES

It's time to talk about The 80:20 Rule as it applies to fitness, weight loss, and weight maintenance. To succeed, you have to choose calories with solid nutritional value 80 percent of the time. This means foods that have a nutritional benefit to them and are often found growing in the ground or on a tree. That is how you love food well. In 1 Corinthians 6:12, Paul reminds us that all things—including food—are permissible. However, not all things—including food—are beneficial.

The same principle applies to other areas of life. We can fill our heads with junk by reading junk books and watching junk on television. Or we can feed our minds with things that will strengthen and enrich us. And with food, the poor quality of what we put in our mouths is often the cause of obesity, disease, and exhaustion. But by understanding how food works and giving your body premium fuel most of the time, you'll lose weight and get fit. At that point you can think about enjoying a hot fudge sundae as a celebration and an expression of gratitude. You can enjoy the occasional splurge because you're now committed to health, fitness, and maintaining a healthy weight. It's fun to eat something you really love occasionally just because it tastes good.

Whether the calories you eat come from ice cream or apples, they all fuel your metabolism. Have you ever heard people explain their weight problem by saying they have a bad metabolism? I used to say it all the time. And here's what I found out: I did have a bad metabolism! Here is why. Because all food ignites our metabolism, think of food as a match. Metabolism is the process our bodies use to break down food and convert it into energy. All weight issues come down to a basic math problem. I was regularly taking in more food than my body could use up. I became overweight by not using all the calories I consumed and then putting even more food into my body. As I put on more weight, my body fat percentage increased. My habitual overeating was sending my body false signals. By consuming more calories than I needed, my body concluded that I was either storing up for the winter or preparing for a famine. My metabolism went into hibernation mode. As I continued to choose to overeat while my body was idle, I became fatter and fatter.

And this is the part we seldom think about: my system needed fewer and fewer calories in order to function, due to all the confusing messages I was sending. My body didn't know how to handle years of overeating and excess calories that weren't being used.

I also put on weight by eating at the wrong time. I would skip breakfast and then gorge on sweets at one sitting. This was hard on my metabolism, since I was fasting overnight and into the morning, in essence slamming on the brakes. Then in one sitting I would overwhelm my metabolism, mostly with sugar. When people say they eat very little and still have trouble losing weight, it's likely they are not only eating the wrong food but are eating at the wrong time.

CALORIES AND WEIGHT LOSS

Just as weight gain is a math problem, so is weight loss. All weight loss comes from a deficit of calories. Period. If you use more calories than you consume, you will lose weight. However, it's important to understand that caloric needs differ from one person to the next.

I have met a few people who have lost a serious amount of weight with gastric bypass surgery. Most of the time they have told me it was the only option left. They had faithfully adhered to every weight-loss plan imaginable and still couldn't lose weight. These folks often believe their bodies are biologically resistant to losing weight. If that were true, why would their bodies not resist weight loss after surgery? Something else must have shifted.

I have witnessed the massive weight loss of many people who have chosen this option, and they have lost weight after the surgery because their bodies have been rerigged to accept and absorb fewer calories. Weight-loss surgery is just a means of forced calorie restriction, not a correction of physiology. The surgical patients were simply forced to consume less food (and fewer calories) versus leaving it up to their willpower and inner strength. Surgery does not overcome or correct the body's resistance to losing weight; it simply limits the body's capacity to consume large amounts of calories.

Please don't think I'm insensitive on this subject. I completely understand the desperation behind the decision to undergo surgery. I seriously contemplated having the surgery myself. Knowing what I know now, I fear it would have caused me to put off dealing with my main problem. I needed to make a personal commitment, no excuses allowed, to choose to live a life of moderation in a world where excess is encouraged. Making such an unconditional commitment to discipline, control, and healthy living is the starting point and the basic requirement for success in fitness and living well. For almost all of us, it is the only way to achieve a healthy balance in life and on the bathroom scale.

Weight Maintenance

Weight maintenance after weight loss is also a math equation. Once you reach a weight range you are content to stay at, you will need to determine the approximate amount of calories it takes for you to remain there. This is based on your age, height, weight, lean muscle mass, and level of activity. I recommend you weigh yourself once a week to stay in check. Based on my usual workout regimen, I can maintain my weight by consuming around 2,200 calories a day. I found this out by paying close attention. For about a month after I had reached a set point for my weight, I calculated the number of calories I took in every day by writing them in a notebook. I also recorded my daily weight fluctuations. (You should keep a similar record.)

At the end of the month, I averaged the totals and concluded that 2,200 calories daily is what worked best. Some days it may be closer to 2,600 calories and some days closer to 2,000. However, as long as the average is the same, my jeans keep fitting. With my exercise program of one hour of intense aerobic exercise six days per week and strength training three days a week, I burn about 2,200 calories a day on average.

Once I was maintaining a healthy weight, I was able to relax a bit on pleasure eating. To make it work practically, I eat clean with no exceptions 80 percent of the time. It's simple and healthy eating, going for maximum fuel from healthy food choices. I eat many of the same foods every day, so I'm already aware of their nutritional content. This frees me from constant calorie counting and the need for frequent decision making. *Should I have the turkey breast or tofu today? What about a slice of cheese if I avoid milk?* Don't wear yourself out with too many decisions. Eating the same thing for lunch every day for a week won't kill you.

Also it helps me avoid the "what am I in the mood for" trap. Deciding in advance what to have for lunch is simple, and it strengthens your self-discipline. As much as possible, I stay clear of foods that are factory packaged. By eating clean 80 percent of the time, I have 20 percent of the time available to eat foods that are imperfectly yummy! By practicing The 80:20 Rule, you can love food and still live very, very well. And you will maintain your healthy weight once you have achieved it.

This works for my body, which is not necessarily an accurate indicator of what your body will do. Remember, you are unique. Many factors determine your daily caloric needs when you are maintaining your target weight.

THE INITIAL PUSH TO LOSE WEIGHT

When you start working to lose weight, you need to further limit your calorie intake. In my first book, *Never Say Diet,* I strongly recommend consuming just 1,500 calories a day while losing weight. Most people who stick to this level can create the necessary deficit to lose weight, as long as they are getting daily exercise. I always use this guideline with clients, and it usually works across the board unless a person has underlying health issues. Diets that encourage drastic caloric restriction—such as 800 to 1,000 calories per day—are nearly impossible to follow. And they often are ineffective because such diets rarely stress exercise.

To burn calories, you must move! Eating five meals a day, each one being about 300 calories, encourages a well-fueled metabolism because of the consistent energy (calories) you are providing to your body. An extremely active person would be the exception. He or she may need a few more calories to avoid going into starvation mode. It's important to space out your meals throughout the day. That is why eating at the right time is a critical component in good nutrition and weight loss.

Here's what you need to know about your calorie needs. Everyone has a set basal metabolic rate. This is the number of calories you'd burn if you didn't move all day. (For example, if you were sick and stayed in bed.) Think of it also as how much energy from food you need in order to maintain all your bodily functions, including growing hair and fingernails.

It's useful to calculate your basal metabolic rate, especially because it helps clue you in to your caloric needs. Having this information will help you judge the number of calories you should be consuming for weight loss and, later, weight maintenance. Use the universally accepted English basal metabolic formula in the box below to determine your basal metabolic rate (BMR).

As you calculate your BMR, recognize that this is just a place to start. You must keep in mind your level of normal daily activity and the additional calories you burn through exercise. This is where it becomes tricky. Everyone burns energy through basic activities and exercise at different rates. Generally,

How to Calculate Your Basal Metabolic Rate (BMR)

Women: 655 + (4.3 x your weight in pounds) + (4.7 x your height in inches) – (4.7 x your age in years)

Men: 66 + (6.3 x your weight in pounds) + (12.9 x your height in inches) – (6.8 x your age in years)

the leaner you are, the faster you burn calories. Also, the more muscle mass you have, the faster you burn calories (compared to someone with a higher percentage of body fat). This makes building lean muscle a priority. Keep all of this in mind as you set a goal for your daily caloric intake.

Finally, you need to pay attention to the ratio of calories you consume from carbs, proteins, and fats. The key is knowing your personal caloric needs and understanding the nutritional value or lack of it in certain foods. For example, fiber contains far less nutritional value but is essential to a balanced diet and to healthy digestion and elimination. The information in the following chapters will help you create a new way of life that involves loving food and living well. You'll understand the properties of food on a deep level. And the by-product can be your making the best choices at the best times.

I watched a *60 Minutes* interview with Olympic gold-medal swimmer Michael Phelps. During the 2008 Olympics, the media couldn't talk enough about how much this guy ate. Reports said that he was consuming from 10,000 to 12,000 calories a day, jamming down fried-egg sandwiches, chocolate-chip pancakes, and entire pizzas in one sitting. Crazy as it seems, an athlete such as Phelps doesn't eat based on nutritional content but on his need for energy. He does eat massive quantities of enriched pasta, and he takes supplements to keep his vitamin and mineral levels in check. Still, he admittedly pays little attention to the quality of what's going into his stomach.

Here's the main difference between this record-breaking swimmer and you and me. Michael Phelps is a young, ultra-endurance athlete with an extremely low body fat percentage. Basically, his "pilot light," his metabolic rate, is always revved, at least while he's training.

Now let's go back to the *60 Minutes* interview. It was just over three months after the 2008 Olympics, the longest stretch Phelps had gone without training. Here is my theory about his eating habits. Sure, Phelps's body was still accustomed to high-calorie meals, but more significantly, his brain was rigged to have the freedom to eat them. During the interview, Anderson Cooper joked as Phelps put away a plate of eggs Norfolk (a variation of eggs Benedict that features Smithfield ham and crabmeat) and an entire cheese quesadilla smothered in sour cream. When discussing the rumors about his eating habits, he said more realistically, "I eat about 8,000 to 10,000 calories"—referring to when he's in training. He told Cooper, "I have to always just constantly shovel in food, because I can lose anywhere from, you know, five to ten pounds in a week."[4] The interesting part was that he admitted to Cooper that he weighs more now than he had ever weighed: 205 pounds. This is more than ten pounds heavier than he weighed at the Olympics one hundred days prior. However, Phelps didn't appear to be concerned. He was planning to be back in the pool the following month and said he would swim off the extra weight.

What does an Olympian's eating habits and calorie intake have to do with the rest of us mere mortals? We live in a world of egg whites and ordering salad dressing on the side. We certainly aren't overindulging in eggs Norfolk for breakfast. Dreaming big, for us, would be having a bagel with regular cream cheese or having french fries instead of a side salad—and on the same day!

But Phelps's story does help us in one area: it sums up the principle of how our bodies operate. Sure, he burns calories at an extremely high level, but this is how it proves the point. The more food we put into our bodies, the more calories we need to use. If we don't use the calories, our weight will increase. This is the same for you, me, and an elite athlete. By the way, Michael Phelps is at an extremely healthy weight at 205 pounds and six feet three inches tall. Recognize also, while energy needs and calorie requirements vary from person to person, the way all bodies add or lose weight is the same. The number of calories you consume versus the calories you burn is the primary math principle to learn. It explains how we lose weight, why we gain weight, and how we can maintain a healthy weight forever.

And if we learn to respect the power of food, we will be free to love it forever.

Carbs: The First Temptation— Go Figure!

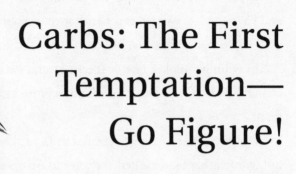

Pasta and Bread, We Love Them! But Don't Love Them Too Much

In the beginning—I'm talking the *real* beginning, at the start of the book of Genesis—there was a man named Adam and a woman named Eve. I'm sure you recall that they are the ones who ate the famous forbidden fruit.

After giving some thought to their dilemma in the Garden of Eden, I had a revelation. It's no coincidence that it all came down to a carb-loaded, tree-born treat, thought by most to be likened to an apple. Sugar was the first downfall for woman-kind!

Some may point out that the problem started with a woman's craving, and I agree. Most women experience strong cravings, especially when coping with PMS. But, remember, Eve didn't have this to contend with—yet. Also, Adam willingly took a bite of the fruit, and he had no menstrual cycle to contend with. They both broke God's command, even if Eve had the idea first.

But get this: the fruit was created by God. The tree it grew on was in the lush garden that God created and gave to Adam and Eve. Then Satan chose to use this sweet treat to trick the first couple into violating God's one prohi-bition, leading to their exile from the garden playground.

Since the Bible doesn't specify that the fruit in question was an apple, you don't have to worry about enjoying a Golden Delicious. But symbolically, we can consider carbs to be a major source of temptation. God created fruit trees and the fruit that grows on them. He made fruit sweet, tart, or tangy—and delicious. Carbs are made in heaven, but they can torture your life like hell! That is another reason we need to study food and its properties and be smart about nutrition and the effects that different types of food have on our bodies.

In the right quantities and proportions, carbohydrates enrich your energy level. But to gain maximum benefit, it's important to know what they are and exactly how they work. Media coverage in recent years has sent "professional dieters" into an uneducated frenzy. With the Atkins diet and many other superlow-carb programs, we have developed an unhealthy fear of carbs. Some people avoid them at all costs. However, when it comes to feeling really good and living well, even controlling our brain function and moods, carbs are very important.

Carbohydrates are the body's main energy source. The body turns carbs into glucose and releases it into the bloodstream. This is how blood sugar is controlled and how you gain the energy to keep your system running well.

The key to making the most of carbs is to understand that there are two types of carbohydrates: simple and complex. Depending on which of the two types you eat, the impact on your body will differ significantly. So it's critical to take this into consideration before you prepare menus for the day's or week's meals.

Simple carbohydrates are also called simple sugars and are chemically made of one, two, or three units of sugar linked together in single molecules. A simple sugar can be just what the name implies: the granulated sugar in your sugar bowl. Things like candy, syrups, and soft drinks are pretty straight-forward examples of simple carbs. They are absorbed quickly into the system. Even better among the simple-carb options are fruit, milk, and yogurt. They are preferable because they contain vitamins and fiber as well as important nutrients, such as calcium.

It's important to remember that you will feel hungry much sooner after eating simple carbs than protein or complex carbs. If you have a fruit-juice-only smoothie or a jelly-filled pastry for breakfast, you may be ready to chew off someone's arm by 10:00 a.m.

Do Snickers Really Satisfy?

You've probably heard the commercial for Snickers bars: "Snickers really satisfies." I wish they would add the qualifier "for about five minutes." Simple sugars give you a quick high, so for a fast boost it does the job. But afterward there is a crash. I remember being at mile twenty of the San Diego Rock 'n' Roll Marathon, feeling like I was closer to death than I had ever been. Of all my experiences with being in a race, this was by far the most difficult. My back was aching, my toes were bleeding, and my legs felt like mashed potatoes.

Our bodies are rigged to go only so far before we come to a halt. When we are engaged in intense exercise, carbs play the most important role. They fill muscles with glycogen, which is the body's favorite source of fuel, especially when it needs quick energy. At mile twenty, my body was letting me know I was running on fumes. This is why, on the night before a marathon, some runners have a pasta party so their muscles can load up for the next day.

In San Diego, just a little more than six miles from the finish line, I hit a wall. I couldn't go on, no matter how hard I tried. I am far from a good runner. People ask how I came to love running, and I am still trying to figure out when it happened. It started as a life achievement. I wanted to accomplish something really, really hard, and running marathons was a way to do that while also raising money for cancer research. (I began marathon training to raise money for the Leukemia and Lymphoma Society because my mom has been battling this disease for more than sixteen years.)

I was three-fourths of the way through the race, and all I could do was try to catch my breath. I'm not exaggerating when I say it was torture. My thoughts were running wild, like wishing they could put narcotics in the Gatorade to numb the pain.

Then, at 6.2 miles from the end, an angel appeared. You can try to tell me that she was a volunteer. But I am 100 percent convinced that God sent one of His marathon angels, dressed her in hospital scrubs at the medic tent, and instructed her to give me a handful of magic. This manna from heaven came in the form of jellybeans! In just a few minutes, my weak and confused body began to perk up. I was able to start running again and finish the race.

Once across the finish line, I smiled as I accepted some bananas, knowing I'd already had my miracle. Jellybean carbs had done their work by giving me quick energy to get a job done.

Know Who the Good Guys Are

Of the two types of carbs—simple and complex—the latter are unquestionably the good guys of the carbohydrate world. Complex carbs such as potatoes are pleasant to the taste buds but not sweet. Remember, simple carbs are one, two, or three units of sugar linked together in single molecules. Complex carbs are hundreds or thousands of sugar units linked together in single molecules. They take longer to kick in after they are eaten, and this is great for supplying long-lasting energy and helping you feel satisfied.

There are two groups of complex carbs: high fiber and low fiber. High-fiber complex carbs are not digestible by humans, because we don't have the enzyme to do the job. (Cows have the enzyme, which enables them to get calories out of grass.) The main stuff in high-fiber complex carbs that is indigestible by humans is cellulose. High-fiber (high-cellulose) vegetables are the healthiest choices for human nutrition, and eating a sufficient amount of these foods is associated with fewer incidents of hypertension, cancer, arthritis, and diabetes. Most complex carbohydrates are high in nutrients and contain plenty of vitamins, minerals, and fiber. Examples of complex carbohydrates include vegetables, bananas, tomatoes, squash, cereals and grains (bread and pasta), potatoes, and rice.

In losing weight, however, it doesn't matter if a carb is simple or complex. After it is digested, it appears in your circulatory system as glucose on its way to the cells where it will be used for energy. So when you're trying to lose weight, the important thing to remember is the way carbs will be used by your body.

Only 45 to 50 percent of your daily calorie intake should come from carbohydrates. Quality is the key, as well as spacing them throughout the day. One gram of carbohydrate contains 4 calories, so let's do the math. Based on a 2,000-calorie-per-day eating plan, 900 to 1,000 calories should come from carbs. This means you should consume 225 to 250 grams of carbs per day.

Unless you are at mile twenty of a marathon or engaged in some other extremely physical exertion, your best carb choice is high-fiber complex carbs. You will feel full longer than with simple carbs. Most of our carbohydrates

Take the Carb Test

Study the following list of carbohydrates, and pick which ones are simple and which are complex. Mark a C (complex) or an S (simple) next to each one. The answer key can be found in the chapter 8 notes in the back of the book.[1] (This is an open-book test!)

orange	Cheerios
croissant	pretzels
oatmeal	strawberries
chewing gum	pasta
grape soda	fudge
cantaloupe	ice cream
bagel	honey
tortilla	dark chocolate
doughnut	saltines

come from cereals and grains, both products of the agricultural revolution. Our bodies are not genetically designed to thrive on large amounts of these processed complex carbs. With the popularity of cereal- and grain-based diets, our carbohydrate metabolism has been upset because we can't handle the large load.

As the pancreas must produce more insulin to keep up with the carbs, more people than ever are becoming insulin resistant. This explains the serious rise in cases of Type II diabetes. Complex carbs with lots of fiber are best when you eat them in their raw state. (Try to avoid processed carbohydrates.) Before a Wheat Thin 100-calorie pack makes it to your home and into your body, it has been stripped of much of its original food value. (You were thinking, *It has wheat. That's good, right?*) Ironically, a whole-grain cracker has little grain left in it.

The cleanest carbs are found in foods that are eaten in their most natural state. The healthiest form of complex carbohydrates is present in high-fiber vegetables such as broccoli, cabbage, eggplant, carrots, and avocados. However, you can spice up your diet in moderation with simple sugars in the form of whole fruits. And include oatmeal, bran, and legumes as staples in your meal planning.

LOVING CARBS AND LIVING WELL

For a lot of us, carbohydrates present the biggest temptation. I am most vulnerable to a warm chocolate-chip cookie. You can keep the potatoes and pasta, but don't hide the sugar from me! So, to get to the place where we can love carbs and still live well, we have to understand how they work and choose the best ones the majority of the time. As you do this, you leave room for the occasional deviation. When a person is just beginning a weight-loss program, it makes sense to remove all simple carbs from one's diet. But only at the beginning.

Avoiding all simple carbs helps to detoxify your body. After a month you'll find that you crave carbs less, and you'll be able to carefully and gradually add them to your meal planning. After eating wisely but not obsessively, your disciplined system will become a new way of life.

The key is in making wise choices and being disciplined, without relying on self-denial, which leads eventually to defeat. I know firsthand that to lose weight and avoid gaining it back, the occasional indulgence is necessary. Not only is it enjoyable to eat food you really love, but it is the only way to counteract the feeling of constantly being deprived. Too much dreaming about delicious food that you can never enjoy leads to diet failure. Typically, it results in binging and gaining back the weight you lost.

I have worked with many carb addicts, starting with myself. If you don't set clear boundaries and stick to them, you will sabotage your diet and fitness program. However, as you act on your commitment to healthy eating, exercising, and living well, you can allow yourself an occasional food celebration. Not only is it earned; it's enjoyable. Your food guilt is gone forever.

Now that we have gotten carbs under control, it's time to study proteins—the power source.

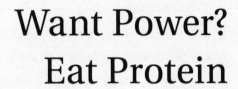

Want Power?
Eat Protein

*Don't Skip the Food That
Keeps You Fueled, Full,
and Feeling Strong*

I am a native South Floridian who
didn't move to a different part of the
country. I conducted a poll of twenty friends and
found that I am one of only two people in that
group who was born in this area. One objection
to living on this peninsula, besides the insane cost
of real estate, is the threat of hurricanes. And let
me tell you, *threat* is the right word.

One of the most memorable was Hurricane
Andrew, which swept across South Florida in

1992. Most of us who are mature can remember where we were and what we were doing when Andrew made landfall. As it blew through, I remember being curled up with my siblings on a twin mattress on the floor, next to my parents' bed. Surprisingly, I was twenty years old at the time.

The few days leading up to the storm also were unforgettable. For a month before the hurricane, my mother had undergone her first chemotherapy treatments for leukemia. Just before the storm was forecast to reach Florida's east coast, my dad and I begged her oncologist to release her from the hospital. She came home, and I thanked God as she lay beside us on a mattress on the floor. As scary as that night was, having mom with us brought so much comfort and peace.

My dad had boarded up our house, but that didn't keep the howling and pounding of hurricane-force winds from reaching us inside. The wind broke off tree limbs that flew through the air and battered anything in their path. The next day our neighborhood was a mess. Trees were down, and miscellaneous items—trash cans, children's toys, basketball hoops—had been deposited in odd places, mostly in swimming pools. All the houses on our block withstood the storm, but only fifty miles away, in Homestead and other parts of Dade County, neighborhoods were demolished. On the news we saw miles of homes that had lost windows and roofs. Tremendous flooding added to the devastation.

While this storm was the second-most powerful of three Category-5 hurricanes that made U.S. landfall in the twentieth century, much of the destruction could have been avoided. I can recall the shocking news from the first reporters on the street after the storm. Many neighborhoods that had escaped the worst of the storm were also leveled. A 1993 report from the Federal Emergency Management Agency cited poor planning, shoddy workmanship, and inadequate building materials as major reasons for the devastation.[1]

Since Hurricane Andrew, many building codes have been rewritten in an effort to prevent such widespread and avoidable wind damage in the future.

BUILDING YOUR BODY TO LAST

The destruction suffered by weak structures in a strong storm is a sobering reminder. No one escapes the storms of life, which is reason enough to power our bodies with the best fuel and to build strength as we lose weight. The foundation of our vitality and health is solid nutrients. Proteins are the building blocks that power every function in your body. The quality of the building materials can make the difference between strength and weakness, energy and fatigue, stamina and collapse. If a storm arrives in the form of a health crisis, this is especially true.

The word *protein* is rooted in the Greek word *protas,* which means "of primary importance." Protein controls all processes of the body, including metabolism. Proteins are essential to a variety of body functions, including the support of our skeletal system. They are involved in the control of our senses, muscle movement, and digestion and in fighting disease. Protein molecules even aid our brain in processing emotions.

According to Elisa Zied, a registered dietician and a spokesperson for the American Dietetic Association, there is no substitute for getting enough protein. "Protein is a critical part of a healthy diet and the right amount helps with everything from higher energy to stronger muscles," Zied wrote. "The trick is to know the healthiest sources of protein and the right amounts for your body."[2] So let's talk about T-bones and tofu.

As I was writing this chapter, I was reminded of the Rocky movies. I even went as far as to watch a video of Rocky Balboa stumbling in the dark to his kitchen and downing five raw eggs. (For the record, the scene was sickening,

111

but I let it slide.) Rocky also let it slide…the eggs, that is! But his message was clear: training to win the fight of his life was the most important thing. I also considered the point made by the scriptwriter. He chose raw eggs as the protein source as a way to drive home the message. The only thing that could have been more intense would have been for Sylvester Stallone to chomp off the head of a fish. I wouldn't have put it past him. This man was going to do whatever it took to get strong. Rocky was using protein exactly in the way it is intended.

Protein is power. Before I give you a gauge for your own needs, let's chat more about power.

How to Eat for Power

Along with fat and carbohydrates, protein is a macronutrient, which means our bodies require large amounts of it. Your body does not store protein, so you have no excess to draw on when the supply runs low. Frank Hu, a professor of nutrition and epidemiology at Harvard University, answered crucial questions about protein in a report he coauthored with Thomas Halton in 2004.[3]

Professor Hu stressed the value of high-protein diets and answered these questions:

- Do high-protein diets increase the rate of the body's ability to burn fat?
- Does a high-protein diet increase a person's sense of feeling full after a meal?
- Does a high-protein diet decrease a person's subsequent energy (calorie) intake?
- Does a high-protein diet lead to weight loss?

His answer for all these questions was yes. The simple explanation is that protein can be converted into glucose for energy. However, the body expends twice as much effort in converting protein to glucose as it does converting carbohydrates or fats into glucose. This is why my marathon angel—the one who revived me with a handful of jellybeans—was not handing out hard-boiled eggs at mile twenty. She knew that for me to get across the finish line, I needed rapid energy-delivering candy. A hard-boiled egg would have taken far too long for my body to convert into usable energy.

If you enjoy steaks, eggs, and cheese, a high-protein diet could be a dream come true. However, eating a high-protein diet should not be a license to ditch sensible food choices. While the enormous fat content in these foods will fill you up, the high saturated-fat content may also lead to clogged arteries. Keep in mind that a diet that is high in protein is measured in relation to other nutrients. As with carbohydrates, one gram of protein is equivalent to 4 calories. I recommend taking in 25 to 30 percent (and no more than 35 percent) of your daily calories in the form of protein.

When planning meals with protein in mind, choose the best sources of protein. Fish, poultry, lean red meat, low-fat cheese, yogurt, and tofu are your best choices, assuming you are consuming protein in the right proportions. Remember that protein is also found in vegetables and nuts. There is nothing essential, nothing life preserving, that we need from carbohydrates. But protein is life preserving because it is broken down by digestion into twenty-two known amino acids, eight of which are essential. Your body must have them, and they can't be manufactured by the body unless you are eating the proper foods. This means we need protein more than carbohydrates for survival.

Every time you deplete your protein supply, the body is forced to feed on itself. Without an adequate supply of protein, the body will break down tissue and muscle. I have seen many elderly people with paper-thin skin and atrophied muscles due to a lack of protein. It may take a little more preparation and planning to incorporate sufficient protein into your diet, but aren't optimal health and longevity worth it?

When I work with clients, I give them an eating plan that starts the day with protein. This is nonnegotiable. It is amazing how many people consume only a small amount of protein from the milk they pour on their cereal. One woman I was training struggled with my protein-for-breakfast rule. She insisted on eating only toast and whole-grain waffles with sugar-free syrup. At the same time she complained of always being hungry and not losing weight quickly enough. While her preferred breakfast menu wasn't a terrible choice, she needed to add protein to maximize strength, encourage weight loss, and cut down on hunger and snacking during the morning. She finally added a protein shake in the morning. (Protein shakes are a great way to get a good amount of protein without too much preparation. The key is to pay attention to the ingredients.)

The first gym I joined was notorious for the awesome protein shakes you could get at the juice bar. David, the creator of these delicious drinks, would come up with something new for me to try every day. I was trying to lose weight and get healthy after tipping the scales at nearly 350 pounds, but I was uninformed about good nutrition. I thought I was having a healthy drink because it came from the gym. The strawberry cheesecake shake still stands out in my mind. It consisted of vanilla protein powder, cheesecake-flavored pudding mix, strawberries, milk, ice, and several large squirts of strawberry syrup. I eventually realized it was around 600 calories, maybe more. This is about double what I should have been having.

You must educate yourself about nutrition, and you have to account for the calories you consume. The best protein shakes come from one serving of soy or whey protein powder. Vanilla protein, a half cup of yogurt, along with a handful of natural fruit and some ice is a perfect choice. A healthy variation is to create a shake with milk, a tablespoon of almond butter or peanut butter, and chocolate-flavored powder. I find that making the same two or three shakes is the easiest way to enjoy some variety while keeping it simple and easy to prepare. (Keep the short list of ingredients handy and in good supply so you don't run out.) Try freezing your fruit and using it to replace some of the ice. And don't forget that bananas are great for this and also provide a good amount of potassium.

The Power of Protein

Protein's power is demonstrated in three ways: building, maintaining, and defending.

- Building: All our body's structural parts (bones, tendons, cartilage, muscle, skin, hair) are made up mostly of protein.
- Maintaining: Enzymes are proteins that speed up chemical reactions in our bodies. Proteins also act as blood transport devices, carrying oxygen to various parts of the body. Blood sugar regulation also relies on protein. Our body's chemical messengers and metabolic regulators—also known as hormones—are made from protein.
- Defending: Protein is used to make antibodies, one of the vital weapons our bodies have for fighting disease.

Let's get back to my client who insisted on eating a breakfast of toast and whole-grain waffles and then complained of being hungry later in the morning. By finally adding a protein shake to her breakfast menu, she started to drop weight rapidly within just a few weeks. Another bonus was that she didn't feel as hungry throughout the day. Feeling fueled and full allowed her to stop picking up extra calories from unnecessary snacking.

It's much easier to get the protein you need if you keep healthy protein foods on hand. Purchase a large package of chicken breasts and either grill them or bake them. My new favorite gizmo is the George Foreman Grill. I really like the cleanliness of this grill and the handy timer control. When you bake or grill chicken breasts, prepare extras and store them for simple recipes such as fajitas. Or you can create a light Caesar salad for dinner. Sometimes my boys will ask for a few grilled chicken strips after school, along with an orange. This is the perfect snack for growing bodies.

Protein helps us build a solid structure, which helps our bodies withstand injury, damage, and weakness. From now on, recognize protein as power. It can keep you full, fueled, and feeling strong!

Fat Is Not a Four-Letter Word

Surprise! You Actually Need It

For most of my life, *fat* sounded like a dirty word. You could've called me a chubby kid while I was growing up. If you had said I was an overweight teenager, I would have been okay with it. And even if you had referred to me as a heavy adult, I might have been irritated, but I could deal with it and move on. But while I never denied that I was overweight, I would have begged you not to ever say I was fat. The mere mention of the word made me cringe.

A funny thing happened recently while I was baby-sitting my three-year-old twin nieces, Taylor and Mackenzie. I watched them prance around with matching ribbons in their hair, sporting matching head-to-toe pink outfits, dancing and laughing. I noticed a recurring theme throughout the day. When I would take one girl to the bathroom, the other needed to go five minutes later, but they never had to go at the same time. It happened again when one of them needed a drink and when one was hungry and pleading for a snack. It was never both girls at the same time. Even the meltdowns over my refusal to give them more M&M's were staggered a bit. Still, these two are the cutest little girls you'd ever meet. Apart from my own kids, of course.

The highlight of our day came during a crisis. Taylor decided to bite her sister on the back while they were arguing over a toy. Mackenzie started to cry. I did my best to calm her down, and when the tears eventually dried, she boldly made a request. "Aunt Chan, we need hot sauce!" She was quite emphatic and then repeated her request. Hot sauce? I thought maybe I had missed the latest edition of *What to Expect: The Toddler Years*. Perhaps it reveals that the newest home remedy for numbing human bites is Tabasco. (This child is only three. There is no way her taste buds crave this fiery stuff just yet!)

I called my mother-in-law to see if she could clue me in, and she did. The twins' mom uses hot sauce to teach the girls a lesson. She puts a tiny drop in their mouths to create a split-second sting. It serves to make them think before they bite each other in the future. Truthfully, I could never have used it on either one of them. After all, I am their Aunt Chan. My job is to paint their fingernails and apply coats of glittery lip gloss.

But the biting incident did get me thinking about other stuff that can serve multiple purposes. It boils down to what you need it to do. In my baby-sitting story, the sauce was intended as punishment. But for anyone who loves spicy food, hot sauce is not generally used for discipline. Adding hot sauce to a burrito can be delicious. Like hot sauce, fat has a purpose. It's an enhancer. It can be delicious and even key to a healthy diet. But overconsuming bad fat can have serious consequences.

A Closer Look at Fat

Fat, as a component in the foods we eat, has a positive, life-enhancing purpose. Most people don't fully understand its value, especially those who have been at war with fat in one form or another, as I was. For quite some time, my nieces will probably think of hot sauce as bad. Similarly, I thought of fat in only one way. I was overweight and was working to lose weight, so the idea of fat was never positive. At that time I also was eating too much of the worst kinds of fat. Eventually I became informed and learned the truth: *fat* is not a dirty word.

Here is the truth: fat is essential to the health of every person. You have probably heard someone say, "She needs a little meat on her bones," when discussing an extremely thin woman. This is because a fair amount of body fat is a sign of health. Fat also symbolizes youth and vitality. Think of the cheeks of a newborn. Don't you just want to squeeze them? It's because they make a baby look healthy. I recently met with a senior citizen group that was having lunch at the beach. The ones that looked the youngest were not rail thin. They also weren't seriously overweight. The few ladies who looked to be only skin and bones seemed much older. Surprisingly, I found out they all were approximately the same age.

A healthy amount of body fat is a good thing aesthetically. Fat also

> ## Ditch the Fat Myth
>
> Some people believe the word *fat* spells out a self-defeating message: if you eat FAT, Forget About Trying (F-A-T) to be thin. This is a myth!

provides insulation and protection for our skeleton and internal organs. In addition, we need fat in the foods we eat for basic survival. No carbohydrates are essential to our survival, but there are essential proteins and essential fats.

Trust me on this. Eating fat can help you lose weight. Say this out loud: "I am supposed to eat and enjoy fattening food." You need to begin saying it without feeling guilty. Here's why: good fats are necessary for living well. By the end of this chapter, you'll know the best fats to eat and the fats to hide from.

KNOW THE ESSENTIAL FATS

According to the Natural Health Information Centre of India, getting the most benefit from fat requires getting enough of the right kind of fat. Fatty acids are a necessary part of your daily food plan. They are found in meat and animal products, but they also are in seeds, nuts, and many other plants.[1] I know some people shy away from nuts because of their calories, but this is a mistake. In fact, nuts are a perfect snack.

Fats are divided into two groups: omega-3 and omega-6. Omega-6 is pretty easy to get into your diet, because it is found in lots of vegetable oils and meats. But omega-3 takes more effort. It can be found in fish (salmon, mackerel, trout) as well as some seeds and nuts, including walnuts, flax seeds, and pumpkin seeds. If you don't consciously incorporate them into your diet, you are probably missing out on the amino-acid benefits from omega-3.

The number-one benefit of omega-3 is enhanced brain function. According to Dr. Artemis Simopoulos, author of *The Omega Plan,* omega-3 fatty acids are undetectable in blood samples of 20 percent of Americans.[2] This should catch your attention, because we're talking about an essential fatty acid. This fat supplies the building blocks for up to half of your brain and also covers every nerve fiber. You can't function well and be healthy without it.

Here is what you need to know about four different forms of fat.

Hydrogenated Oils

These are the fats to avoid. They basically are fats that are produced by adding hydrogen to an existing molecule. In that process, unnatural fat is created. This is why you need to avoid hydrogenated oils and trans fats as much as possible. All nutritional value of the original oil is lost in the processing, and the resulting by-product of these oils is added shelf life for packaged foods and a toll on your arteries. Hydrogenated oils are more challenging for your body to break down. They travel sluggishly through your arteries, and they can slow down the flow of blood and cause blockages. Check for hydrogenated oils on food labels. Nearly every box on the cookie aisle lists this kind of fat.

Vegetable Oils

Don't let the word *vegetable* throw you off. While many oils come from vegetables, not all of them are healthy. While olive oil is beneficial, corn and sunflower oils have fewer positive effects. Generally, vegetable oils are what we use for baking cakes, making salad dressings, and deep-frying. Stay clear of vegetable oils that come in a solid form. Margarine and shortening are hydrogenated vegetable oils. In contrast, olive oil has the most benefits for good heart health.

Saturated Fats

This fat is most commonly found in red meat. Heart disease has been recognized since the 1940s, and eating too many saturated fats is a big contributor. Ironically, hydrogenated vegetable oils also were introduced in the 1940s. Today, heart disease is the number-one cause of death in the Western world. Saturated fat is not the only culprit, of course. In moderation, this form of fat is acceptable. Everyone loves a hamburger now and then.

As with any food, moderation and keeping nutrients in proper proportion is a key. No more than 10 percent of your daily intake of calories should come from saturated fats. Saturated fats lack double bonds between the carbon molecules of the fatty acid chain. This means they are fully saturated with hydrogen atoms. Too much of this fat will cause heart and artery blockage. High proportions of saturated fats are found, not just in red meat, but also in dairy products such as ice cream, butter, and cheese. And due to saturated fats, limit your intake of coconut oil, cottonseed oil, palm kernel oil, and chocolate.

Cholesterol

Contrary to popular opinion, cholesterol is not from the devil! It is a natural fat and a versatile compound that, in small amounts, is vital to the proper functioning of your body. Cholesterol is responsible for producing hormones such as estrogen and testosterone, and it occurs in high concentrations in the brain and nervous system. Most of the body's cholesterol needs are met through the cholesterol produced by your liver from saturated fats. The remainder of the cholesterol comes from the foods you eat, such as egg yolks and some seafood such as prawns. Remember to have your cholesterol levels checked by your family physician annually. Heart disease can sometimes be prevented by monitoring the high-density lipoprotein (HDL) and low-density lipoprotein (LDL) levels of cholesterol in your blood.

Remember that fat calories should make up about 25 percent of your daily total, and allow no more than 12.5 percent to come from saturated fats. One gram of fat is equivalent to more than double the number of calories contained in a single gram of protein or carbohydrate. However, you don't need to eat very much of it to feel full.

When you learn to do the math, you'll find that it's much easier to keep the amount of fat in your diet at a healthy level. If you need to consume about 2,000 calories per day to maintain a healthy weight, then 500 calories should come from fat (all forms combined). This means no more than 250 (one-half) of the calories should come from saturated fat.

One gram of fat contains 9 calories. So to calculate the calorie content of the fat in your diet, multiply nine times the amount of fat, in grams, that you eat in a meal. For example, if you're eating 10 grams of fat, you're getting 90 calories from fat (9 calories x volume of fat consumed in grams = calories from fat).

In a healthy diet, you derive no more than 25 percent of your total calories from fat. If you are consuming 2,000 calories per day (from all types of food), your daily meal plan should include no more than 500 calories from fat (25 percent of the daily total). This translates to approximately 55 grams of fat per day. No more than 27 of the fat grams (one-half of 55) should come from saturated fat.

Don't forget, loving food well leaves room for a T-bone steak and a slice of Key lime pie, just not every day. Also, if you happen to enjoy food with a kick, don't come asking me for the hot sauce!

Do the Math on Calories from Fats

We'll use 2,000 calories per day as an example of your total daily calorie intake. To calculate the recommended calories from fat per day, use the following guidelines.

No more than 25 percent of your combined daily calories should come from fat. So begin by multiplying your daily combined calories (2,000) by 25 percent (.25): 2,000 x .25 = 500 calories from fat per day.

Now, calculate how much fat you should eat each day to supply 500 calories. Divide 500 calories by 9 (the number of calories contained in a single fat gram): 500 ÷ 9 = 55.56 grams of fat.

To calculate the limit on saturated fat in your daily meal plan, multiply your total daily calories (2,000) by 12.5 percent (.125): 2,000 x .125 = 250 calories.

To calculate the grams of saturated fat needed to produce 250 calories, divide 250 calories by 9 (the number of calories in a gram of fat): 250 ÷ 9 = 27.78 grams of saturated fat per day.

How to Make Meals Meaningful

Use The 80:20 Rule to Give Mealtimes Purpose Every Day

*A*ll food has meaning, not just the special foods we enjoy as part of a celebration. Since food is essential to life, and the right combination of food maximizes your energy and strength, every meal has meaning. Food takes on additional meaning when you understand how calories work and how to maximize the benefit of food by preparing it in certain combinations. Meal planning and preparation is the time to use your creativity.

Since meaning is closely associated with purpose, every time you put food in your mouth, it should serve a purpose. Most of your meals will be about getting the right amount of good carbs for energy and then adding lean protein for strength and throwing in a little healthy fat.

Food also has meaning when it is part of a bigger celebration. For me, Thanksgiving is the best holiday of all. I enjoy doing the cooking and trying new recipes. I can get quite irritated when my family starts grabbing plates and scarfing down the food without saying a proper blessing.

Several years ago my mother began a new Thanksgiving tradition. We now go around the table and tell something we are thankful for, and then we say something nice about the person to our right. It becomes part comedy show and part cryfest. (Last year my daughter Ashley said to her sister, Kayla, "I'm glad you stopped stealing my friends and got your own.") My sweet Pepa, who was in his eighties, continued to thank the Lord for always being true and faithful. Thanksgiving won't seem the same this year since Pepa has now passed on to meet the Lord, where he can thank Him in person.

Thanksgiving is special, and expressing our thanks makes the meal meaningful. But the day wouldn't mean as much if we followed the same rituals throughout the year. Likewise, the special foods on the table at Thanksgiving aren't what we should eat every day. But on Thanksgiving, when we thank God for His goodness and share what we appreciate about one another, food really does take on extra meaning.

FOOD THAT IS MEANINGFUL EVERY DAY

The great news is that occasionally food should be for feasting! We can celebrate our blessings and thank God for the pleasure of eating. Throughout history, eating rich foods was reserved for special times. It made an event special. We don't feast every day, of course, but at every meal, food needs to be meaningful.

As we learn the nutritional benefits of different types of food, it's clear that the food at most meals should satisfy the needs of our body, not our brain. We don't eat for entertainment but for fuel. The secret to making every meal meaningful is not to allow your schedule to control your mind. Eating is not designed to be recreational, to distract you when you're bored, to comfort you, or to be a friend when you're lonely. Food has one primary purpose: to fuel your body. Food supplies the energy you need to live well.

To keep food meaningful but not in control of your life, shift your thinking about the food you eat. By committing yourself to this discipline 80 percent of the time, you free yourself to celebrate the remaining 20 percent of the time. So prepare your mind in advance, which will set your expectations. A full 80 percent of the time, all the food you consume should accomplish the following:

- supply vital nutrients
- satisfy your hunger
- deliver long-lasting energy

These three rules apply without variation 80 percent of the time. There is no room for compromise or negotiation, which is much of the value of The 80:20 Rule. To get the fuel your body needs while losing weight, becoming fit, and getting strong, your eating has to be disciplined. The only way I have found to maintain my weight is to have these rules in place. I know in advance that for specific time periods and for most mealtimes (eight out of ten), I adhere to these three rules. There are no exceptions. I never allow myself to order a piece of cheesecake if I eat out on a Monday. I can avoid cheesecake on Mondays because I know there will be opportunities later on to have cheesecake or some other dessert.

The 80:20 Rule does not give you an excuse to be undisciplined. You eat clean, without exception, 80 percent of the time. This limits calories, maximizes the value of the food you eat, and promotes weight loss. What helps you commit fully to this discipline is the knowledge that the other 20 percent of the time you can splurge—within limits.

Here are the food rules for the remaining 20 percent of the time. By maintaining strict control eight times out of ten, you can relax a bit 20 percent of the time, when food should

- offer an opportunity to be creative
- satisfy a food-related desire
- give you the freedom to celebrate and indulge

The reason that many strict, take-no-prisoners approaches to dieting fail is the sense of permanent deprivation. You still have to live in the real world, and your friends, relatives, and colleagues won't suddenly stop celebrating with food just because you are committed to getting fit and losing weight. With a hard-core diet, you end up going to birthday parties, engagement parties, going-away parties, and anniversary celebrations only to watch everyone else enjoy cake, hors d'oeuvre, punch, and those yummy mini-quiches. How can you join the celebration when you have your hands on nothing more festive than a cup of water and six celery sticks?

GETTING THE MOST FROM THE 80:20 RULE

In my book *Never Say Diet,* I showed how you can reserve limited opportunities for splurging. As I've worked more with clients, I've found that it's helpful to be more specific about allowable times of celebration and indulging. That's why I now recommend The 80:20 Rule. When you know in advance that your new way of life promises regular opportunities to enjoy a favorite dessert or a special meal, then the majority of your life—when you are sticking to your calorie limit every day—becomes more doable.

One reason dieters fail to limit their calories is that they allow themselves to reconsider their level of commitment. They allow for too many menu options 100 percent of the time, rather than only 20 percent. But by sticking to The 80:20 Rule, your menu choices and meal planning are never in limbo. You don't have to waste time wondering, *Should I or shouldn't I?*—a guessing game that gets you into trouble.

I want to set you free from the ordeal of struggling with food and decisions about food. After all, living well includes being free from the things that used to defeat you. Trust me, no one ever plans to gain weight after losing it. Yet I have stopped counting the number of times I have heard the same story from all sorts of clients. Regardless of their personal circumstances or age or social status, the story ends up the same. Complacency is the culprit. They bought one too many excuses and then found themselves in a downward spiral, with their self-control and good intentions disappearing like water down a bathtub drain.

I have been there myself. I would set a goal, and sometimes when I achieved it, I would ask, "What happens next?" It has happened to all of us.

Think about sports for a minute. When a team makes it to the top, whether it is the World Series, the Super Bowl, a collegiate national championship, or the World Cup, fans immediately wonder if the team can do it again. But when it comes to weight loss, you don't want to need to do it ever again, right?

Your Goal Is Living Well, Not Losing Weight

To avoid losing weight and then gaining it back and feeling like a failure once again, shift your focus from dieting to your life as a whole. The point is to live well, not to fit into a certain size dress or to weigh what you did in high school. Yes, you want to lose weight, get fit, build strength, and maintain a healthy weight for a lifetime. But don't settle for just changing your body; commit to becoming the best you can be: body, mind, and spirit.

When I weighed nearly 350 pounds, I was desperate to lose weight. But losing 200 pounds was just the by-product of the changed life I desired. I knew that my body was not a separate part of me. In order to lose weight and get fit, I realized I needed a complete life change. In fact, that was what I desired from the start. You can't change your life by continuing to do the same things you did before.

When your primary goal is to be the best you can be, you don't achieve that goal in a year or two. In fact, you truly won't reach this goal until you get to heaven. I started on my quest for a new life in 2001, and it led to dramatic changes in all areas of my life. But have I achieved my goal? Not by a long shot. I'm still not there. Nearly ten years later, I continue to set new goals all the time. One is to love food and live really well. Living well includes my health, but not just body health. I want to live well in mind and spirit also.

Losing weight is a big part of the overall goal, because failing in this area holds us back in other areas. So reaching your target weight and then maintaining that weight becomes one of the first goals you will set. And it's possible to achieve that goal when you allow food to have purpose and meaning. I will never forget this proverb: "Ask a rich man how much money is enough, and most times the answer is 'just a little bit more.'" If you always feel that you need to lose just a little more, even after you have achieved your healthy target weight, it will destroy your efforts to change your life. It is the reason you and I have suffered in the past when trying to find a balance in our relationship with food. Becoming fit and living well is a process that will last the rest of your life.

APPLYING THE 80:20 RULE TO YOUR DAILY LIFE

To get the most from The 80:20 Rule, decide first how you will allot the 80 percent and the 20 percent. When allocating the disciplined 80 percent of your everyday life, use your lifestyle to guide you. The approach that works best for me is to think in terms of the week as a whole. But at the beginning, I did it differently and suffered as a result.

For a few years immediately following my weight loss, I would consider 20 percent of the time to be basically from Saturday afternoon to Sunday night. This was my time to indulge in an eating frenzy of whatever I felt like. The other days—from Monday morning to midday Saturday—I ate a restricted amount of calories so I could save them for the weekend. That means that all week long I had no sugar, no junk, and very small portions. That means I went to bed feeling hungry and deprived five nights a week. Still, I did maintain my weight doing this. My emotions, however, were still out of whack when it came to food. Having this much freedom for the entire weekend would send me into the next week feeling bloated and depressed. I had a big psychological letdown on Monday morning, knowing I wouldn't allow myself to have even a bite of chocolate for the next five days.

I would eat too many calories over the weekend, knowing I was approaching another five-day restriction period. This is why cheat days are a bad idea for people who have cheated with food too often in the past. As you rethink your eating habits using The 80:20 Rule, don't approach the ratio with large blocks of days in mind. Instead, spread out the times when you maintain your discipline and the times when you are free to splurge.

I recommend thinking, not in terms of complete days or weekends versus weekdays, but in terms of a single twenty-four-hour period. If you are eating five meals per day of 300 calories each, for instance, make one of the five meals a fun meal. This does not mean losing control, as if you're sidling up to a Las Vegas buffet line. I simply mean that you should make one meal a day more pleasurable than the others. You still concentrate on solid nutritional content in your meal planning, but you do it more creatively. And part of being creative is fitting good nutrition into your normal day, not the opposite of scheduling your life around food.

I think in terms of what's going on in my life that particular day. For example, if I know my husband and I will be meeting friends for dinner, I will hold back some calories from my other meals. This will give me more freedom to indulge at dinner. Looking forward to eating something in the future also makes a little hunger during the day more manageable. A sense of anticipation about a future meal actually helps you practice complete self-control 80 percent of the time.

Love Food with Creative Meal Planning

By following The 80:20 Rule, you stick to your daily calorie limit 80 percent of the time with no exceptions allowed. Keep in mind, as I said before, long-term weight management requires that you pay attention to the bottom line: calories. But you can succeed in this disciplined approach because you know you will have the freedom to splurge on occasion. And because food has a valid purpose and meaning, it's important to be creative in your meal planning. You also should want to serve your family meals with purpose.

All foods should serve the first three purposes I discussed earlier:

- supply vital nutrients
- satisfy your hunger
- deliver long-lasting energy

To eat the best food for maximum energy with the fewest calories, incorporate carbohydrates, protein, and fat (all three) into your meal planning. Here is how it works. Build most of your meals by incorporating complex carbohydrates, protein, and healthy fats. Keep reading and you'll find examples of meals that do all of this. The recipes later in this chapter give you a healthy nutritional balance, plus they taste really good. They all offer vital nutrients and will satisfy your hunger. In addition, they deliver long-lasting energy. I promise that if you plan meals by paying attention to vital nutrients, satisfying your hunger, and providing long-lasting energy, you will stay the course of weight management for a lifetime. By the way, all these recipes are simple and easy to prepare. It should take you no more than fifteen minutes to put a meal together.

TIPS TO MAKING BREAKFAST MEANINGFUL

Be sure to begin your day with protein. There are no exceptions to this. Protein satisfies you for a longer period of time compared to carbohydrates alone, which keeps you from feeling starved by midmorning. Protein also promotes the building of lean muscle. Don't forget that a Harvard study reported that people who skip breakfast are four times more likely to be overweight than those who regularly eat breakfast.[1]

Don't hesitate to adjust the seasoning or certain ingredients in the following recipes to satisfy you or your family. Just keep track of the nutrients and calories. Having a repertoire of four or five breakfast meals that are healthy, quick, and simple to prepare will reduce the temptation to pick up a dough-nut at the office.

Cheesy Breakfast Burrito Olé

1/3 cup Southwestern Style Egg Beaters
1 slice Fat Free Kraft Singles
1 whole-wheat tortilla
1 tablespoon salsa
low-fat sour cream (optional)

Spray the pan lightly with nonstick cooking spray, and cook the scrambled Egg Beaters. When the eggs are almost done, tear the slice of cheese into pieces and mix it into the eggs. Place the mixture into a warmed tortilla, and add salsa before folding it up. Add a dab of low-fat sour cream on top if you'd like.

   Nutritional information: 1 burrito has approximately 140 calories, 3 g fat, 15 g carbs, 20 g protein

Apple Cinnamon–Pecan Oatmeal

(Yields 6 servings)
3 cups rolled oats (old-fashioned)
2 teaspoons baking powder
1/2 teaspoon salt
2 teaspoons ground cinnamon
2 cups low-fat milk
1 large egg, beaten

$^1/_3$ cup applesauce

$^1/_4$ cup melted butter

$^1/_2$ cup brown sugar

2 cups chopped apples (red works best)

12 tablespoons chopped pecans

6 teaspoons honey

Prepare a rectangular baking dish with a light coating of cooking spray. Preheat oven to 400 degrees. In a large bowl, combine the rolled oats, baking powder, salt, and cinnamon.

In a separate bowl, mix together the milk, egg, applesauce, butter, and brown sugar. Stir both mixtures together and pour into the baking dish.

Bake for 20 minutes.

Then fold in the chopped apples, and bake 20 more minutes until the top is lightly browned. When finished, spoon into serving bowls and top each serving with 2 tablespoons of chopped pecans and drizzle with one teaspoon of honey.

Nutritional information: A 1-cup serving is approximately 277 calories, 8 g fat, 39 g carbs, 8 g protein

TIPS TO MAKING LUNCH MEANINGFUL

Having a solid lunch will prepare you to end your day with a smile. Also, I have found that many people attempting to lose weight have the tendency to be overly hungry in the late afternoon. In paying close attention to my clients' meal choices, I often find their lunch selection was too sparse. Keep lunch hearty enough that you won't binge before dinner but not so heavy that you

require an afternoon siesta. In allocating calories to different meals throughout the day, lunch is the best time to add extra calories. This is because you
still have several hours of being active to burn them off.

"Meet Me in the Mediterranean" Wrap

(Yields 4 wraps)

2 medium zucchini, about $1/2$ pound each, sliced lengthwise and then
        laterally into $1/4$-inch slices

2 tablespoons olive oil

$1/8$ teaspoon salt

ground pepper, to taste

1 cup hummus

4 pieces whole-grain pita bread

$1/4$ cup pine nuts

2 large tomatoes, sliced

2 cups baby spinach leaves

$1/2$ cup sliced red onion

4 tablespoons mint

Preheat the broiler. Discard the outermost slices of zucchini and brush
the rest with oil. Dust with salt and pepper. Place on a baking sheet
and broil about three inches from the heat for 5 minutes on each side
or until tender and slightly browned.

Spread $1/4$ cup hummus on each wrap, and sprinkle with 1
tablespoon pine nuts. Top with a few slices of tomato and zucchini,
$1/2$ cup spinach, a few slices of onion, and 1 tablespoon mint. Roll up
and cut in half on a diagonal.

Nutritional Information: 1 wrap is approximately 340 calories, 9 g of fat, 42 g of carbs, 16 g of protein

Terrific Tuna Salad

(Yields 6 servings)

2 6-ounce cans chunk light tuna, drained

1 15-ounce can small white beans, such as great northern, rinsed

10 cherry tomatoes, quartered

4 scallions, trimmed and sliced

2 tablespoons extra-virgin olive oil

2 tablespoons lemon juice

$1/4$ teaspoon salt

$1/2$ cup fat-free mayonnaise

freshly ground pepper to taste

Combine tuna, beans, tomatoes, scallions, oil, lemon juice, salt, mayonnaise, and pepper in a medium-size bowl. Stir gently. Refrigerate until ready to serve. Serve with whole-grain crackers, whole-wheat bread, or pita pockets.

Nutritional Information: per serving, 253 calories, 8 g of fat, 20 g of carbohydrate, 31 g of protein

TIPS TO MAKING DINNER MEANINGFUL

Your dinner menu should always include protein. Add a salad or veggies and a small portion of complex carbohydrates. At my house we grill chicken about three nights a week. I serve it with a bit of barbecue sauce or maybe a dash of garlic and lemon-pepper seasoning to jazz it up. Alongside is usually some steamed broccoli or a big salad. There may also be half a sweet potato with a tablespoon of brown sugar and cinnamon or brown rice and a ladle of black beans on top. As you might expect, my family occasionally gets bored with this, so they beg for something else. Here are a few healthy dinner recipes everyone enjoys.

The Perfect Shepherd's Pie

(Yields 4 to 6 servings)

1 pound 90% lean ground round

1 cup chopped onion

2 cloves garlic, chopped

1 14.5-ounce can diced tomatoes with green peppers and onions, undrained

1 1-pound package frozen mixed vegetables, thawed

1/2 cup fat-free, low-salt beef broth

2 teaspoons dried Italian seasoning

1 teaspoon salt, divided

1/2 teaspoon freshly ground pepper, divided

11/2 pounds baking potatoes, peeled and cubed

1/3 cup 2% reduced-fat milk

Preheat oven to 375°. On the stovetop, cook the beef, onion, and garlic in a large Dutch oven over medium heat until the beef is browned. Drain. Stir in tomatoes, vegetables, broth, Italian seasoning, 1/2 teaspoon salt, and 1/4 teaspoon pepper. Bring to a boil. Cover, reduce heat, and simmer 10 to 15 minutes, stirring frequently. Spoon beef mixture into a 2¹/₂ quart casserole dish coated with cooking spray.

Place potatoes in a large saucepan, cover with water, and bring to a boil. Reduce heat and simmer, uncovered, 15 minutes or until very tender. Drain well and return the potatoes to the saucepan. Mash well. Add the milk and the remaining salt and pepper. Mix until smooth. Spread the mashed potatoes on top of meat mixture and bake for 20 minutes or until thoroughly heated.

Preheat broiler. Broil casserole 5 minutes or until potatoes are browned.

Nutritional Information: per serving, 443 calories, 8 g fat, 69 g carbohydrate, 29 g protein

The Yummiest Chicken Chili

(Yields 6 servings.)
8 chicken breasts, 4 oz. each
¹/₂ teaspoon salt
¹/₂ teaspoon pepper
1 15-ounce can pinto beans
1 15-ounce can dark red kidney beans
1 15-ounce can light red kidney beans
1 15-ounce can black beans in sauce
2 15-ounce cans tomato sauce
1 onion, chopped
1 cup mushrooms, chopped
2 cloves garlic, chopped
chili powder to taste

Boil the chicken in water, salt, and pepper for one hour over medium heat. Drain off the water, and shred the meat with a fork. Next mix in all the beans (undrained) and the tomato sauce, and add chili powder to taste. Add the onion, mushrooms, and garlic, and then let the chili simmer over low heat for another hour.

Nutritional Information: per serving, 365 calories, 3 g fat, 44 g carbohydrates, 27 g protein.

PART 4

Getting Strong—Inside and Out

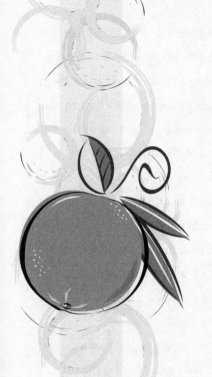

Today, Get Your New Life Moving

To Live Well You Have to
Change Some Daily Habits

I know I won't be winning any popularity contests with this chapter. But no matter what, I have to tell the truth. Ready?

Exercise is as important as brushing your teeth.

If you can't buy this, then you'll never experience the deal of a lifetime. To live well while loving food means you have to get moving. We are all made to move. It's a natural part of living, not an inconvenience or something to dread.

If you don't believe me, think about the magic that happens when you walk. Your legs and arms work together to propel you in a forward motion. We are designed to do it. Once when I was taking a brisk wintertime walk in New York, I found myself clinching my hands in my coat pockets to stay warm. But with my hands stationary, and my arms not involved in my forward motion, my pace slowed way down. Try it some time.

When you limit or stop the motion of the upper part of your body, it drags down the effectiveness of your leg motion. In contrast, when you get arms and legs moving in tandem, working together, it's magic! The National Center for Health and Statistics says Americans don't get enough exercise. According to their findings, only 26 percent of adults engage in vigorous exercise three times per week.[1] This statistic is troubling. It means that 74 percent of the adult population is not exercising regularly.

Many of the e-mails I receive that mention working out strike a similar note. People tell me they just can't seem to find the time. Finding the time to do anything that we value is a challenge, given the demands of our schedules and our hectic pace of life. Time is a precious commodity. It is also one of the few things we all possess in an equal amount—the same number of hours every day. It doesn't vary according to age, gender, geography, or marital status.

Since we're dealing with just twenty-four hours, you need to know a few essential things to make exercise happen. First, you don't exercise just so you can lose weight or lose it more quickly. Exercise is not something you force yourself to do for just a while, that is, until you achieve your target weight. On the contrary, exercise is as important to your health as good nutrition. It's impossible to live really well if you stop exercising once you have achieved a healthy weight. It would be like saying, "I'm going to stop taking showers because after that last one I finally got clean." Do you want to eat tomorrow? Then you'll need to exercise.

THE ESSENTIAL STEP OF SURRENDER

Last year I ran a contest on my Web site. I wanted to find a few special people I could connect with who felt they could use some one-on-one coaching from me for a month via e-mail and weekly phone chats. I sent out an e-blast and asked for stories of personal struggles, and I received hundreds of responses. After going through them all and praying for God to help me with the decision, I chose two special women. After selecting the winners, I learned that one of them, Carmen, lives only an hour from my home. I want you to read the highlights of her story.

Hi, Chantel:

I began my Brain Change on March 31, 2008, after spending my spring break reading your book and feeling for the first time in a great many years like I had hope again. I was desperate to lose weight and, more importantly, transform my lifestyle to never be overweight again.

By my Brain Change anniversary (March 31, 2009), I was down 85 pounds. (My beginning weight was 275 pounds; my present weight is 190 pounds on a 5'1", 47-year-old

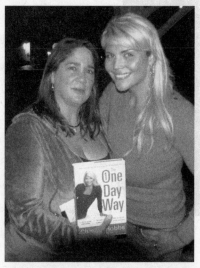

Carmen, left, lost eighty-five pounds in one year and is still losing. Chantel showed up for a surprise visit to give Carmen a copy of Chantel's book *The One-Day Way.*

body!) I am amazed at how I have transformed my life, my looks, my health, and most of all my belief system that I will never be on a diet again and that I will always feel and look my very best. I love your motto "progress, not perfection," and that is the way I live my life now. I have also been able to inspire friends and co-workers.

Carmen asked me to help her amp up her program. She felt like getting time with me would provide a renewal of energy. I chose her for one reason: her perspective. She understood that I am not a weight-loss superhero fashioned to save her and the world from the fat trap. Instead, she had taken my personal story, advice, and encouragement as it relates to faith, food, and fitness and applied it to her life. She was not putting pressure on me to do the impossible. Instead she was asking me to support her at the mental and emotional crossroads she was now facing. To me, this was a win-win situation. I would be able to help Carmen stay the course through prayer and by giving her a fresh perspective and exercise tips. In return, she would be reminding me of God's unique will for my life to be a walking testimony to the world and through it to share His love.

I let Carmen know she was a contest winner, and we began our correspondence. During the course of the month, she lost another ten pounds. She also found out how to make exercise a greater priority. Best of all, we've established a friendship I believe will last for years to come. Carmen represents exactly why I feel commissioned by my Savior to write books, speak, and share each day.

GETTING THINGS GOING

Once you decide that you will never go back to the way things used to be, it's useful to have practical ways to build new habits into your daily life. Here are a few of the most doable, useful, and practical ways to find time to exercise.

Don't Let the Day Get Away from You

There are reasons that life gets out of control. One is that life, by definition, is unpredictable. So things are going to come up that you haven't planned for. The other leading reason is that we fail to plan for the things we can predict.

For example, you can predict that life will crowd out the things that you don't make a priority. So to succeed in making exercise a part of your daily routine, do it first thing in the morning. Set your alarm to go off forty-five minutes earlier. You might even consider wearing your exercise clothes to bed, just to catch an extra few minutes of sleep. Or if you are cost-conscious, approach your exercise schedule as you would a dentist appointment. If you break it, you pay a financial penalty. (Put five dollars in a jar when you miss a workout. Then use the money that accumulates to start a fund for a smaller pair of jeans.)

Make Your Exercise Plan Doable

Depending on your personality and temperament, you might feel that if you can't do something perfectly, it's not worth doing. Or you might tell yourself that if it's worth doing, it's worth pushing yourself to the breaking point right from the start. Or maybe you think of exercise as torture and conclude that you might as well choose a form of exercise that you hate, since you'll hate it for the rest of your life, no matter what happens.

I have some advice for you. If exercise were intended to do you harm, I wouldn't devote my life to helping you and others make it a regular part of your life. Furthermore, exercise doesn't have to be daunting or frightening or even something you dislike. When you begin an exercise program, you ease into it just as you would if you were learning a language or training for a new career.

Exercise doesn't always need to be long and intense to be effective. Remember this: the most effective exercise is the one you do every day. The key to beginning an exercise program is to get moving. You can build up gradually to more intense workouts. But if you never start moving, you'll never exercise.

Change Happens Only When You Start Doing Things Differently

People who accomplish great things are successful because they did the hard things it took to bring about change. As a working mom, Carmen had to fit in exercise after work. We all have responsibilities and deadlines to meet and too many demands on our time. However, there are things we must fit in every day—brushing our teeth, for instance. Likewise, exercise needs to be part of the daily essentials.

Once Carmen decided to make the changes that would deliver the life she desired, she had to find the time to make it happen. Exercise was non-negotiable, and she was ready to make the necessary sacrifices. Maybe Carmen could have lost weight by starving herself on a diet of 500 calories a day. This would be the calories she would be burning at the crack of dawn. But taking weight off with deprivation requires tremendous dedication, which is where Carmen had struggled. She wanted a lasting life change, so she made a commitment to get moving. And once she started, she found that she felt better physically. There is an immediate reward to exercise, even in the first stages before it gets more demanding.

Match Your Daily Schedule to Your Goals

Most people who are inconsistent with exercise complain of feeling tired and weak. Or they say they run out of steam early in the day. Don't let the initial fatigue and muscle soreness stop you. Schedule regular exercise into your day, and keep at it. In order to synchronize your desires with your life, you have to change your daily schedule.

As you get started, commit to at least five days a week of cardio exercise with at least thirty minutes per session. In later chapters I will give you exercises to do, not only to get started, but to kick up your exercise once you master the basics. I also will introduce you to the perfect workout partner. And in chapter 15, "You Were Made to Move," you'll find exercises that will help you feel firm for a lifetime.

These are things you may have dreamed of for a long time. Now is the time to start making them happen. So schedule it and then stick to your schedule. No excuses allowed.

Make Your Top Goals Your Top Priority

Do you know someone who is a big football fan? My husband, Keith, is a huge Miami Dolphins fan. Every September, on the day of the first regular season game, Keith has to find a place to watch the game no matter where we are that Sunday or what we are doing. Seriously, any football widow will know what I'm talking about. And he isn't happy unless he is coaching the players (which is what he thinks he's doing from our family room). But if we can't be home at game time, he goes to Plan B. Once we were at a wedding, and Keith somehow found a television. A few years ago we rented a house in the mountains for a week, and my crazy husband brought our satellite dish and installed it when we arrived. (I'm serious!)

Here's what I know. Keith cares deeply about the game and the outcome, every single time. He wants to watch it when it happens. He doesn't want just to read about it the next day or hear about it from friends who saw the game. Keith has an emotional investment in the team. If they win, he celebrates. If they lose, I go shopping, because I don't like to see his disappointment.

If you're a huge fan of any sport, television program, or summer concert series, you understand my husband's willingness to go out of his way to be a part of the NFL season. Exercise can become that sort of thing in your life.

You can reach the point where other things will be put off, delayed, or rescheduled so you can get in your daily exercise. In fact, for you to live well, exercise has to be given that level of priority.

A New Life Is Worth the Sacrifice

If you have ever learned to play a musical instrument, worked hard to develop a new skill, or perhaps gone back to school to earn an advanced degree, you know that making a change in your life requires sacrifice. You don't accomplish anything important by chance. You apply energy, concentration, effort, and commitment. So now, as you make the deal of a lifetime, answer these questions:

- Are you so committed to a new life that you are willing to drop your old habits?
- Do you have an unwavering and motivating emotional attachment to the deal of a lifetime?
- Are you prepared to go to extremes, if necessary, to make your new life a reality?

As Carmen learned, the only way to change her life was to get rid of her old excuses. I have never heard anyone say, "Well, once I figured out I really have no time to work out, I just decided it was fine to stay overweight."

I have vivid, painful memories of the tears I shed when I was morbidly obese and losing hope that my life would ever change. Now, more than ten years after accepting the deal of a lifetime, I would never trade my hour in the gym each day for those desperate tears.

You can choose to never go back to a life of pain and frustration. Don't trade the deal of a lifetime for the old life of disappointment and defeat. Start your new life now by doing what you were made to do. Get moving.

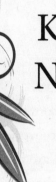

Keep Exercising, No Matter What!

Even When Circumstances Change, Make Sure You Keep Moving

*J*ust when you find something that really works and you start to settle into an exercise routine, get ready to change it. It's not that you want to give up a preferred type of exercise or abandon your regularly scheduled time slot. It's just that life keeps changing. Things come up all the time that seem to undermine your planned routines.

When that happens, and I guarantee it will, be flexible. The worst thing you can do is allow a shift in your work schedule, added family demands, or some other unforeseen circumstance to interrupt your exercise program. So build on your commitment to keep moving by adding a commitment to be flexible, adaptable, and resourceful. You can learn important lessons from the interruptions and challenging circumstances that life brings your way.

The Value of Humility

Humility is a virtue that we would all like to possess. But wouldn't it be nice if we could develop it without discomfort or inconvenience? The trouble with humility is that you don't learn it through favorable circumstances. It is learned most often through difficulty and hardship.

Humility often develops out of our looking like a goofball in front of others. When it becomes obvious to everyone around us that we're flawed, it's humbling. We also learn about humility in difficult life circumstances. In some situations we feel completely out of control, whether in a crisis or just doing life and dealing with one curve ball after another. When we realize that we're powerless to help someone, to solve a problem, or to relieve someone's pain, it's humbling. As much as we want to help, we often are not able to.

The other side of humility is its power. Humility gives us the freedom to adjust when life doesn't go exactly the way we planned. And that seems to be most of the time, doesn't it? Genuine humility involves developing the attitude that honestly says, "I don't know everything. I'm the last person who has it all together, but I am willing to learn."

I have gotten a dose of practical humility in connection with physical pain. Take, for example, the time I decided to prove I was special by running two marathons only three weeks apart. That's a combined 52.4 miles. Many people can run one marathon a month, but two? That's just crazy talk! So I decided I would do it. I trained, I ran both races, and I did finish. But afterward I wondered why.

My mother-in-law, Linda, is famous for saying, "You might get what you want but not want what you get." This could never have been truer for me. I finished the second race in horrific pain. Tendonitis in my Achilles haunted me for the next six months. What was I thinking when I decided to enter both races?

With all the pain I suffered, you might think I had learned my lesson. But, surprisingly, the following year I again decided to run two marathons, and once again they were only three weeks apart. That time I wanted to prove to everyone that I had advanced in my athletic training.

During the second race, I became extremely dehydrated. There I was in the Palm Beaches Marathon, and I had to beg a stranger to run inside her house and bring out some table salt. If she hadn't, I'm convinced I would have ended up in the emergency room. Talk about a humbling experience. The woman looked totally puzzled when I staggered up to her, asking for some Morton's.

I should have kept the table salt incident to myself. But later I felt the need to defend the extended time it took me to finish the 26.2-mile course, so I told my family about it. I guess you could call this selfish humility. My family saw right through my story, reminding me that I was nuts to do two marathons again so close together. As if I might have forgotten it, I had to admit, "I don't have it all together, and I'm really not all that good!"

The craziest part is that I shouldn't have been caught off guard by the catastrophe on this day. I know from experience that I get dehydrated faster than most people. I was sodium depleted from the humidity and my excessive sweating. Also I had been overtraining and felt exhausted going into the race. Stupid, stupid, stupid! It wasn't like I didn't know better.

Most recently, I injured my foot: some silly flareup of one of the nerves on the bottom, between my first and second toes. This time I hadn't done anything extreme. I was just doing normal things, but the pain was still aggravating. At first I took an over-the-counter pain reliever and went on my merry way. I kept running, Spinning, and doing other exercises that put a lot of pressure on my foot. But the pain would return with a vengeance immediately after the anti-inflammatory wore off. Still, exercise is a part of my daily life. If I were going to quit because of a little pain, I would soon be contemplating a boycott on brushing my teeth or taking showers. I wasn't going to give up exercise just because my foot hurt.

I was in a predicament. I needed to find some exercises I could do that avoided putting more stress on my foot. And they had to be exercises that I wouldn't hate doing. There is nothing worse than an exercise program that you really, really hate.

Love Exercise and Live Well

When you launch a new exercise program, begin with exercises that fit your life as it is right now. I truly love Spinning, so the idea that I needed to shift to a different exercise that would spare the impact on my feet was not a welcome prospect. Still, the important thing is to keep moving, so I adjusted.

I considered all the options. When I need to find a new exercise, I opt out of salsa and step aerobics. When I've tried these in the past, I've held up everyone else who showed up for a real workout. I'm the chick the teacher has to stop to help every ten seconds. I have come close to causing major collisions during the grapevine move that aerobics classes are famous for. According to my husband, I would do best to keep my dancing talent a secret. In other words, he thinks I should dance only when no one else is looking.

So after I hurt my foot, I found I could get a great workout on an elliptical machine. It's actually relaxing and puts less pressure on my foot, and I still sweat a bunch. I can increase my intensity while listening to some great music, and it gives me a chance to forget about deadlines and laundry.

I have even taken up fast-paced walking. In the beginning this was a bit humiliating in light of my marathon running. Check this out, though. I have found an unbelievable, perfect walking partner. My Partner has never stood me up and has never been even a moment late. Also, He doesn't complain about anything—ever. Instead, we just talk about what's going on in my life. The encouragement He gives me is awesome. I really think I could walk forever when we are together. When the workout is over, I feel like a new creation, His creation.

God is the best workout Partner and Companion of all time! And He wants to be yours too.

Don't hear me wrong: Chantel the marathoner hasn't switched to mall walking. I walk at a fast pace and sometimes bring weights to increase my heart rate. Or if I'm on a treadmill, I adjust the incline to add more challenge. Normally I wouldn't use a treadmill, but trying to find a decent hill in South Florida is impossible.

GET READY FOR A CHALLENGE

The key to any workout is to be challenged. Once you get used to a certain intensity level, it's essential that you vary and increase the intensity. Our bodies become accustomed to a given work load. If your goal is to burn a significant number of calories, your workout must always remain a challenge. The goal is not to get comfortable with an exercise but rather to continue to increase the intensity. To improve heart health and blood flow, your efforts need to be amped up regularly.

I have seen people at the gym on the same StairMaster year after year with the look of "I couldn't be having more fun if my tooth were being pulled without Novocain." This should never be you! Your workouts should not feel monotonous.

Here's how to avoid both monotony and the tendency to get comfortable with the same workout. What exercise can you do that will present a challenge but that you can also enjoy? My husband loves to play basketball. It's a great workout. My daughters love cheerleading—another great workout. My sister-in-law Kristen was a swimmer in high school. When she joined the gym awhile back, the lure was the Olympic-size pool.

Whatever exercise you choose, you must leave room for life. There may be an unforeseen illness or injury, a schedule shift, or changes in your financial situation. So be open to changing your exercise routine even after you find a program you really love.

Recently a woman cornered me in the grocery store and mentioned she had read my book *Never Say Diet*. She told me she was a previous gym rat—someone who works out for hours at a time. But recently she had lost her job and could no longer afford the gym dues. She confessed that she had stopped exercising because she lacked access to a gym. But it doesn't have to be that way. There are many ways to work out that don't involve going to a gym. What changed for her was not the ability to exercise but the convenience of exercising the same way she had in the past. She needed to readjust and reorganize.

To lose weight and change your life, you have to reject excuses. If you hurt your foot, as I did, or if you have to save money by dropping your gym membership, find ways to exercise that accommodate your new circumstances.

Ann and her husband, Lou, moved into the house next door about the same time we moved into ours. I've never met people more Italian than this couple. They're both really cool! As I sit in my office most days, I look out the window and see Ann gardening. I have been the recipient of her homegrown tomatoes many times. With all the work this takes and the cost of fertilizer and everything else, Lou jokes that these tomatoes are worth about twenty bucks apiece. But for Ann this is about fulfillment, not finances.

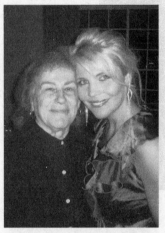

She has also turned gardening and yard work into real exercise. Ann will take a plastic bag from the grocery store, and one by one, she'll pick up all the leaves the wind blew on to her lawn overnight. It can take her an hour or more to do this each day. I've overheard Lou beg her to let him rake them up. Her response is, "And me, uh, do what? Watch television all day?"

My neighbor Ann, who doesn't let anything prevent her from staying active. She does yard work and keeps a garden, sharing homegrown tomatoes with others.

Wow! Ann gets what more people should understand and practice if they really want to get control of a weight problem. She knows, "Hey, I'm still breathing. I can move, and I get to do something that I love each day!" Ann also isn't bound by limitations of age or circumstances. This is a beautiful lesson for us all.

14

How to "Bring It" with Interval Training

The Guaranteed Way to Get Maximum Results from Exercise

*K*erri is my closest friend. If you ask her where she's from, she won't hesitate to tell you, "L.A." Just don't assume it's the L.A. where movies are made and earthquakes threaten. The L.A. she's talking about is Lower Alabama. She's part redneck and part beauty queen, but most of all she's fully lovable.

Kerri's most endearing quality is the enthusiasm she shows when she's really excited about something. And trust me, it doesn't take much. The two of us can make standing at a grocery store deli counter into a laughfest. Recently she tasted a slice of lunchmeat and nearly did a backflip because she thought it was so delicious. I had to tell the woman working behind the counter, "Sorry, my friend doesn't get out much." Whenever I need encouragement, Kerri is the first person I call—especially when I'm writing and need someone to listen to my work.

When she thinks I'm onto something big, she has a great saying. She'll stop me midsentence and blurt out, "Bring it...bring it..." with a full Southern twang and even sweeter intentions. My friend is letting me know I'm seriously nailing it.

If Kerri were a fitness program and not the world's finest friend, she would be interval training. We've already talked about the need to be flexible and adaptable with your exercise regimen. If you find a form of exercise you enjoy and it feels right, that's great. But if you only engage in the same form of exercise and never vary the intensity, you won't get the maximum benefit from your efforts. Even if you vary the length of time you spend exercising, you still need to vary the intensity also.

Interval training helps you "bring it!" like nothing else. You can nail your workouts every time, and isn't that what you've been wanting? Interval training needs to be a part of your regular cardiovascular exercise routine. I promise, this form of training is going to keep you on the right track to losing weight, being superfit, and feeling strong. It kicks up your cardio routine and helps maximize your workout time.

Intervals are based on a very simple concept. You begin with a light warmup, then you increase and decrease the intensity level over specified time periods. The duration of these time periods should vary from one exercise session to the next. Basically, intervals help train your heart muscle to perform at maximum efficiency.

WHY YOU NEED INTERVAL TRAINING

If you really want to live well, you have to include interval training in your fitness program. Here are five reasons:

- Interval training speeds up your metabolism even when you aren't exercising.
- Interval training is the best conditioning possible for the heart muscle.
- Interval training will help you break through a plateau in your weight-loss program.
- Interval training takes less time than cardio sessions that are done at a steady pace.
- Interval training is challenging and fun.

Interval Training Speeds Up Your Metabolism

When you limit your cardio exercise to a fixed pace, your body eventually adapts to that level of intensity. At first, exercising at a steady pace delivers benefits. It burns calories while you are doing it, so it has an important place in your exercise regimen. However, if you always exercise at the same pace, you will miss out on the best benefits that exercise has to offer. That's why I am so high on interval training, which prevents your body from adapting to an established pace of exercise. This is because the intensity level is constantly increasing and decreasing. This forces your body to work harder to keep up with the challenges you are giving it.

After you complete an interval workout, your body will need more time to recover. This causes an after burn, which is the time frame when your metabolism is revved to replenish the oxygen in your bloodstream. Technically, this is called your energy post-oxygen consumption system (EPOC). This process makes you burn lots of calories after your workout ends and, at the same time, speeds up your metabolism.

Interval Training Excels at Conditioning the Heart Muscle

All cardiovascular exercise is great for conditioning the heart muscle. However, interval training has a special benefit. During the workout you are increasing the blood and oxygen flow in incredible amounts before backing off and then repeating the heightened intensity. Because the blood and oxygen flow is highly intense, the heart muscle meets a healthy challenge in learning to respond. All muscles get stronger with added intensity. When bodybuilders train, they add more weight to their sets to develop stronger muscles. The same principle applies when you want to create a superstrong heart.

Interval Training Can Help Break Through a Weight-Loss Plateau

After you have worked with your fitness program and lost weight—but haven't yet reached your target weight—you often will find that the pace of weight loss slows to a near standstill. You may have lost fifteen pounds in the first eight weeks and then find that you can lose only three pounds over the next six weeks.

What happened? If you have been using the same exercise regimen during that time, a weight-loss plateau is not surprising. The solution is interval training, because when you vary the workout plan, it helps create a positive confusion for your body. After having adjusted to your standard, repeated exercise regimen, suddenly your system has to readjust. The rebound can cause an increase in your metabolism. When you have hit a plateau, try a few new interval sessions to force a breakthrough.

Interval Sessions Take Less Time Than Steady-Paced Cardio Exercise

How would you like to spend less time working out but get better results? I'm in! How about you? This is what high-intensity interval training provides. Because of the intensity, you could never keep at it for extended periods of time.

If you have watched Olympic sprinters, you know they run the race of their lives in no more than twenty seconds. On shorter sprints, the athletes run for less than ten seconds. Listening to interviews with some of the competitors even a half hour after their race ended, I could still hear them working to breathe. They could never run at that speed for long periods of time. Sure, I understand we're talking about elite athletes. But even for the rest of us, as we raise the intensity of our workouts, we can spend less time working out.

Interval Training Is Fun

Getting on the same treadmill, day in and day out, and setting it to 3.5 miles per hour can get really boring. The great thing about interval training is the excitement of setting new challenges for yourself. Intervals are versatile. You could create a new one nearly every time you work out. Intervals also have the potential to be fun, especially as you begin to experience greater results with less time invested.

HOW TO GET STARTED

You should incorporate high-intensity intervals two times a week, with regular cardio at least three times per week. Don't do intervals every day, because your body needs a chance to recover in between. And remember, you should

How to Monitor the Intensity
of an Interval Workout

INTENSITY LEVEL ON A SCALE OF 1 TO 10	DESCRIPTION OF EXERCISE INTENSITY
1–2	"I'm beginning to move, but I can't wait until this is over."
3	"Just another day in paradise. I'm feeling pretty good."
4	"This is getting hard, but it is so worth it."
5	"Hey, working out is fun!"
6	You're beginning to feel invigorated. Moderate effort
7	"This isn't so fun anymore!" Moderately intense
8	"Why are my legs burning?" Intensity builds significantly. You couldn't maintain this level for an extended period.
9	"Whoa. I need to catch my breath!"
10	"All out, no-holds-barred work effort."

HEART RATE IN BEATS PER MINUTE (bpm)

Your heart rate is increasing slightly.

Heart rate is up to 65 percent of your maximum. (If your maximum is 120 beats per minute, this would be 78–80 bpm.)

Your heart rate is 65–75 percent of your maximum. (If your maximum is 120 beats per minute, this would be 78–90 bpm.)

Your heart rate is 75–80 percent of your maximum. (If your maximum is 120 beats per minute, this would be 90–96 bpm.)

Your heart rate is approximately 80–85 percent of your maximum. (If your maximum is 120 beats per minute, this would be 96–102 bpm.)

Your heart rate is 85–92 percent of your maximum. (If your maximum is 120 beats per minute, this would be 102–110 bpm.)

Your heart rate is at least 92 percent of your maximum. (If your maximum is 120 beats per minute, this would be 110 bpm or higher.)

push your limits each time. Don't be surprised if you feel more exhausted later in the day after interval training.

Later in this chapter I'll give you three thirty-minute, varied interval sessions that you can mix into your workouts. Of course, after you get the hang of it, you can create your own. Please consider wearing a heart-rate monitor. This serves to keep a close check on your body's response to exercise. During interval training your heart rate should be elevated to no higher than your maximum heart rate. (See the information at the end of this chapter to calculate your maximum heart rate.)

As you set out to complete an interval workout, it's important to monitor the intensity of the exercise. The effort and exertion are measured in terms of percentages. Monitor your level of exertion on a scale ranging from 1 to 10. For a standard guideline, refer to the scale on pages 164–65. Even better, use a heart-rate monitor so you will have an accurate and constant reading on your heart rate.

Most standard cardiovascular activities are suitable for an interval session. The key is to raise and lower the intensity several times throughout an exercise session, using the level-of-intensity guidelines you just read. Following are three suggested interval workouts. Each one is different in order to provide variety and to strengthen your heart. Time durations and intensity levels are given for each interval. Adapt the three interval workouts to fit your favorite cardio exercises.

- jogging/running/sprinting
- walking on a treadmill and adding an incline or faster pace
- stationary bike, adding speed and resistance
- elliptical, adding speed
- swimming, adding speed

Interval Session 1: "Fire It Up!" (30-minute session)

Begin with a five-minute warmup at levels 1–3 (consult the chart "How to Monitor the Intensity of an Interval Workout," pages 164–65), then continue:

Minutes 1–5	warm up to level 5
Minute 6	level 8
Minute 7	level 9
Minute 8	level 5
Minute 9	level 8
Minute 10	30 seconds at level 9 and 30 seconds at level 5
Minutes 11–13	level 6
Minute 14	level 7
Minute 15	level 8
Minute 16	level 9
Minute 17	level 5
Minute 18	30 seconds at level 9 and 30 seconds at level 5
Minute 19	level 7
Minute 20	level 8
Minutes 21–23	level 6
Minute 24	level 7
Minute 25	30 seconds at level 9 and 30 seconds at level 5
Minute 26	level 7
Minute 27	level 8
Minutes 28–29	level 6
Minute 30	30 seconds at level 9 and 30 seconds at level 5

Recover at levels 5, 4, 3, 2, 1 for several minutes until your heart rate drops below 50 percent of your maximum.

INTERVAL SESSION 2: "LET IT BURN" (30-MINUTE SESSION)

Begin with a five-minute warmup at levels 1–3, then repeat the following interval two times.

Minute 1	level 8
Minute 2	30 seconds at levels 4–5; 30 seconds at level 9
Minute 3	levels 6–7
Minute 4	45 seconds at level 8; 15 seconds at level 9
Minute 5	30 seconds at levels 4–5; 30 seconds at levels 6–7
Minute 6	levels 1–3
Minute 7	30 seconds at level 8; 30 seconds at level 9
Minute 8	level 5
Minute 9	level 6
Minute 10	level 9
Minute 11	30 seconds at level 6; 30 seconds at level 7
Minute 12	30 seconds at level 10; 30 seconds at level 5
Minutes 13–14	levels 6–7
Minute 15	30 seconds at level 9; 30 seconds at level 5

Repeat for another 15 minutes.

INTERVAL SESSION 3: "GO FOR IT, THEN RELAX" (30-MINUTE SESSION)

This is twenty minutes of interval exercise followed by ten minutes of exercise at a steady pace. Begin with a three-minute warmup at levels 1–3.

Minutes 1–3	levels 1–3
Minute 4	30 seconds at levels 6–7; 30 seconds at level 8
Minute 5	level 9

Minute 6	30 seconds at level 10; 30 seconds at level 5
Minute 7	level 8
Minutes 8–9	levels 6–7
Minute 10	level 8
Minute 11	level 9
Minute 12	30 seconds at level 10; 30 seconds at level 5
Minute 13	levels 4–5
Minute 14	level 8
Minute 15	level 9
Minute 16	levels 6–7
Minute 17	30 seconds at level 8; 30 seconds at level 9
Minute 18	30 seconds at levels 1–3; 30 seconds at level 5
Minute 19	30 seconds at level 10; 30 seconds at levels 6–7
Minute 20	15 seconds at level 8; 15 seconds at level 5; 30 seconds at level 9
Minutes 21–30	steady state cardio at level 8

How and Why to Use a Heart-Rate Monitor

I have heard too many clients say, "I don't need to wear a heart-rate monitor. I check my pulse sometimes, and I know where I am." It's no coincidence these are often the same people who say they exercise regularly but don't notice continued results. Plainly, if Lance Armstrong needs a heart-rate monitor, so do you.

The monitor is like having a map to track your body's response to exercise. The gadget helps you maximize your workout by showing you exactly how intensely your body responds to exertion during exercise. I prefer the Polar brand, and I feel that the most accurate monitors use a chest strap and a watch.

Research has shown that as you grow older, if you maintain a decent level of fitness, your maximum heart rate doesn't decline. Therefore, in line with my training and experience, I teach the Karvonen method, which requires a little effort to calculate. However, it is usually much more accurate than other methods.[1] To begin the calculation, it is best to wear a heart-rate monitor to bed. As soon as you wake up, record your resting heart rate. Do this a few days in a row (five is ideal). Then take an average by adding the numbers and dividing the total by the number of days you kept the record. Then fill in the blanks that follow, using the Karvonen method.

Here is the formula: 220, minus your age, minus your resting heart rate, multiplied by the intensity percentage (refer back to "How to Monitor the Intensity of an Interval Workout," pages 164–65), plus your resting heart rate, equals _____. This number is your target heart rate at that level of intensity. Once you calculate your target heart rate (bpm) at different levels of exercise intensity, you will have reliable numbers to use during interval training. Before you fill out the six levels of intensity below, arrive at your starting-point number, which is 220, minus your age, minus your resting heart rate: _____ (referred to in the formula below as "your number"). Use this number to complete the following calculations.

Now fill in your target heart rate at six levels of intensity, from warmup to the top level.

Your number, times the intensity level (percentage goal), plus your resting heart rate, equals the number to use for target heart rate.

_____ x .50 + _____ = _____

_____ x .65 + _____ = _____

_____ x .75 + _____ = _____

_____ x .80 + _____ = _____

_____ x .85 + _____ = _____

_____ x .92 + _____ = _____

15

You Were Made to Move

Getting Back to the Ball

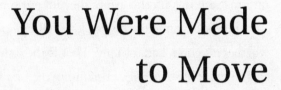

lients and friends ask me all the time to give them the best exercises for tightening this or strengthening that or shrinking something else. Frequently they are concerned about a "bat wing," the excess skin that dangles below your arm when you raise it.

I wish there were a secret list I could share with you that could fix every concern you have with your body. But I have studied this for years, and I've found that the real secret is this: there is no secret! I sometimes browse the magazine aisle at the drugstore and look through the ones that are specifically geared toward women. The hype related to how to get the best results from exercise is hilarious. Do people really think it's possible to get serious abdominal definition after having three kids and being thirty pounds overweight for the past ten years? Sure, sometimes the articles contain great information. But at other times they fill our minds with empty promises.

You didn't come to this book for false hope or lies. You want the truth whether it's good, bad, or ugly. That is the only way you can live well in all areas of your life. Aiming at becoming the best we can be will motivate us to get the maximum benefit from strength training.

All the exercises I teach in this chapter are effective, but they won't completely fix every problem area. Will they give you the flattest tummy in the world? Perhaps, but that is not always possible to achieve. Can they help you build lean muscle and feel stronger and tighter? Yes, absolutely! Can they deliver a healthy spine and improve your posture? Guaranteed! Will they also deliver a considerable improvement in your physique? One hundred percent! There's the real truth, friend.

So if you can handle the truth, let's go for it! Training with a stability ball is fun and challenging.

WHY USE THE BALL?

If you read my first book, *Never Say Diet,* you are familiar with the stability ball. If you haven't read it, don't worry. You and the ball will soon become great friends. To really live well, you will need to establish a long-term approach to keeping all the muscles in your body conditioned. Incorporating a stability ball into your regular routine is great for many reasons. The ball is round, obviously, which creates imbalance. When you use the ball to sit on or to put your feet on while doing strength training, you are doing much more to challenge a greater number of muscles. The ball's instability also causes you to develop agility and coordination. Even your toes get a good workout. When trying to maintain proper form and balance while doing a move, all the abdominal and back muscles will become engaged. As a busy wife and mom, I get excited about doing workouts that will deliver the best results while cutting down on the time I spend doing them.

What's All the Chatter About Core Strength?

You may wonder about all the talk surrounding the core. Why concentrate so much on muscles that seem to be secondary? The biggest reason is that the muscles at our core are anything but secondary. They support everything else.

The intense stress our bodies are under with financial pressures, hectic schedules, and relationship maintenance takes a serious toll. As a result, a lot of people have developed a seriously weak spine. And let's not forget, the neck and shoulders are notorious for holding our tensions. The core muscles are at the center of it all, since the spine is designed by God to connect all the muscles in the body. Also, the rise in the amount of time people spend sitting at a computer and watching television has created a boatload of individuals who complain of lower-back issues and chronic pain.

These are common, serious complaints. And the solution for almost all of us is to strengthen the muscles at our body's core. All the muscles in the lower back, for example, are supported by the core muscles. When people dream about having nice abs or a "six-pack," they're thinking about the largest, strongest, and most superficial abdominal layers. I see the same people in the same spot in a gym doing the same abdominal curls or sit-ups. By doing these movements exclusively, they are limiting their movement to a forward-bend motion.

To give you a well-balanced and complete workout, which includes core muscle strength, I designed fifteen new exercises. These will give you the most complete, overall strength-training workout. And you can use them for the rest of your life. They are meant to help you progress over time, going from a beginner level to intermediate and eventually to advanced status.

The best part is that all the exercises can be made more challenging. By increasing the length of time you hold a movement and adding to the intensity with heavier dumbbells, your workout can be constantly revived and refreshed! Adding more repetitions is also a good way to create a new challenge. Feel free to add variety and higher levels of difficulty as you see fit. However, be sure to pay close attention to your form by using the demonstration photos provided with the exercise descriptions. And don't forget to have a stability ball!

YOUR PERSONAL STRENGTH-TRAINING PROGRAM

If you want to see results, you need to do strength training at least two times per week. The ideal timing is before you do your cardio workouts. No matter what, aim to get to the point where your muscles achieve failure by the end of each set. This means you can't do another repetition or hold the move for more time without compromising your form. The all-time greatest mistake people make with strength training is quitting too soon. As a result, they don't see any change.

By pushing yourself to the point of failure, you strip muscle fibers. This repair process is what causes muscles to rebuild even stronger. In turn, you also become leaner. Don't forget, fat is mushy and expandable. It takes up much more space under the skin than hard, sleek muscle.

I'm a strong proponent of weight training for women. Don't worry that you might get too big or bulky. Physiologically, it just doesn't work that way.

It is impossible for a typical woman to suddenly sprout huge muscles. It takes the right genetics and proper nutrition in the correct ratios, plus significant rest versus work effort, to cause muscles to respond with serious growth. However, men can grow big muscles in a relatively short period of time because they have a much greater amount of testosterone. So don't worry, ladies!

All the exercises described in this chapter can be done in one session, or you can incorporate them into a few workouts, depending on your comfort level. The cool part is that you won't need expensive equipment or a gym membership, just a stability ball and a few sets of dumbbells. Each exercise targets all the major muscle groups.

I recommend using free weights rather than a weight machine. When you use a weight machine, your body is supported by the equipment, which allows many of your muscles to do nothing during an exercise. In contrast, when you use free weights, you involve many more muscles for stability and support as you do the movement. Using free weights allows you to get even more benefit from the exercises.

As you begin a strength-training program, maintain a training log to chart your activity and progress. This also reminds you of the day's workout plan. It's a good idea to look back regularly and note your improvement. A spiral notebook works well. A log is also available as a download on my Web site, www.faithfoodandfitness.com. For additional strength-training exercises, check out my books *Never Say Diet* and *The One-Day Way*.

EXERCISES TO GET YOU STARTED

If you are new to strength training, you are probably unfamiliar with using a stability ball. While I understand that you may be a bit intimidated and nervous, get ready for a challenge! Here are five exercises especially for you.

Standing Side Bend

What's happening: This movement will stretch the entire upper torso of your body while strengthening your back muscles.

1. Take hold of the ball and raise it to chest height while standing with your feet a little more than hip-distance apart. Turn your feet outward and bend your knees slightly.

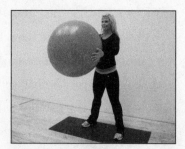

2. Lift the ball overhead while keeping your arms straight.

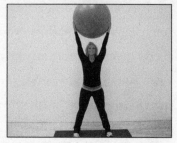

3. Bend to one side. Count to five slowly, then return to the starting position. Each time you complete the movement, try to increase your range of motion a bit more. Bend to the other side and again count to five. (Your goal is to bend low enough to each side that your torso and head are level with your waist.)

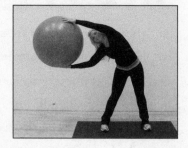

Do three sets of ten repetitions on each side. With each set, try to hold the position a few more seconds. Working up to fifteen seconds per repetition would be awesome!

Lunge Rollouts

What's happening: This movement will tone and strengthen your hip flexors, hamstrings, and quadriceps.

1. With the ball on the ground beside you, stand in a lunge position with about two feet of distance between your front foot and back foot.

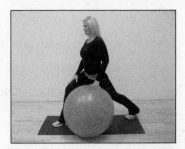

2. While placing your hand on top of the ball, move the ball in front of your back leg. Next drop that knee toward the ground.

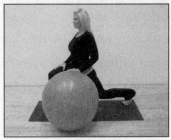

3. As you hold this position, roll the ball about one foot forward with your hand.

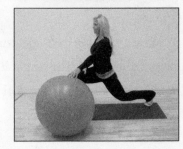

Continue the exercise, completing three sets of fifteen repetitions on each side. Try to take only a fifteen-second break between each set.

Sumo Squats

What's happening: While looking like a sumo wrestler is probably not your main objective, this movement will strengthen your inner thighs, buttocks, and quadriceps.

1. With the ball in hand, take a wide stance. Your feet will be spread about one foot out from your hips on each side. Next turn both feet out.

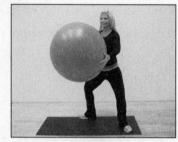

2. Raise the ball overhead and bend your knees so you begin to squat.

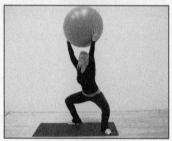

3. While holding the squatting position, lower the ball to chest height and count to five. Return to the starting position.

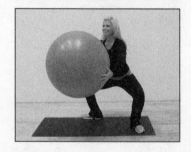

Continue squatting for three sets of fifteen repetitions. You will burn more calories by keeping your heart rate up during the exercise. Do this by taking only a fifteen-second break between sets.

Wall Roll-up

What's happening: This exercise will challenge your hamstrings primarily. It will also strengthen your entire abdominal region.

1. Lie on your back with the ball close to a wall. Bend your knees and raise your feet in front of you, propping them on the ball.

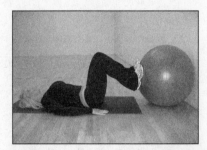

2. Using your entire lower body for power, roll the ball up the wall by pushing with your feet. Eventually you will raise your hips off the floor.

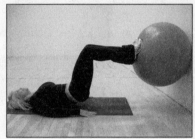

3. Be sure to walk the ball up the wall until you have extended your legs and there is only a slight bend in your knees. At the top, hold the position for ten seconds. (Be sure to keep your shoulders flat on the ground.) Then return to the starting position.

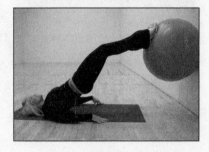

Repeat the roll-up for three sets of ten repetitions.

Alternate Leg Extensions

What's happening: You will feel this movement in both your upper and lower body. However, this exercise is especially good for creating definition and firmness where the buttocks and legs connect.

1. Lean forward with your chest resting on the ball and your knees bent and on the floor.

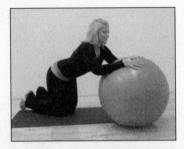

2. Straighten one leg out behind you so that only the top of the foot is touching the ground.

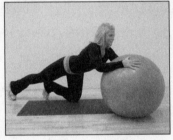

3. While pointing your toes away from you, lift the straightened leg so your foot comes off the floor. Raise the extended leg until it is even with your hip.

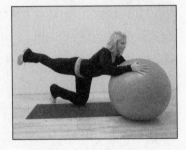

Return to the starting position and repeat with the other leg. Do this exercise for a total of two sets of ten repetitions on each side.

EXERCISES FOR INTERMEDIATE STRENGTH TRAINING

Hooray! You are ready to move on to exercises of greater difficulty. Not only is this exciting, but it also indicates that your body is becoming stronger and more acclimated to doing harder exercises. Add the following five exercises to your workouts, and don't be afraid to push your personal limits.

Straight-Leg Side Lift

What's happening: This will really work on your outer thighs, oblique muscles, and entire upper body. At the same time you will be challenged to balance your body.

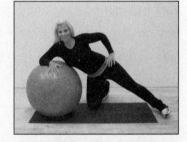

1. With one knee on the ground, hug the ball into that side and extend the opposite leg straight beside you. Your hand on that side should rest on the hip of the extended leg.

2. Reach up and straighten the arm on the side that is extended.

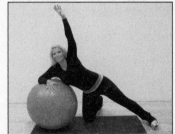

3. Holding this position, use the other arm to roll the ball away from your body until that arm is fully extended. Hold this position for ten seconds.

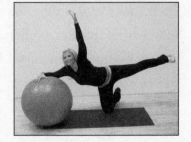

Complete two sets of ten repetitions on each side.

Bent-over Biceps Curls

What's happening: Besides toning your biceps, you also will strengthen your lower back. (You will need dumbbells for this exercise.)

1. Kneel on the floor with your chest resting on the ball, thighs against the ball. Come up on the balls of your feet. Extend your arms over the ball in front of you and hold the dumbbells straight out with your palms up.

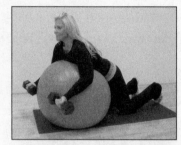

2. Lift your knees off the floor and straighten your legs behind you. Your feet will remain bent on the floor. Raise your chin slightly and curl the dumbbells up toward your shoulders. Concentrate on squeezing the biceps muscles.

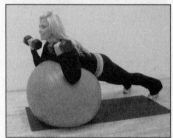

3. Lower and repeat.

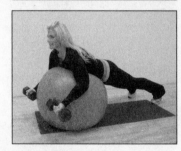

Do this for a total of three sets of ten, twelve, and fifteen repetitions. Using a set weight for your dumbbells is a good way to start. Begin with a light weight, perhaps five-pound dumbbells. Eventually, though, you will want to increase and vary the amount of weight you are using.

Bent-over W-Back Squeezes

What's happening: Your posture will improve greatly with this movement. Also, you will tone and strengthen your upper, middle, and lower back. (You need dumbbells for this exercise.)

1. Lie with your chest on the ball and your stomach and abdomen pressed into it and your legs extended behind you. Pick up the weights at each side, beginning with your arms hanging straight down toward the floor.

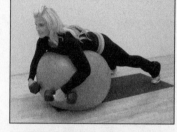

2. Pull the weights up, using your shoulders, while raising your chest off the ball and pressing your upper thighs into the ball. Next, lift your arms and bend your elbows. Imagine forming a W with your arms and back. Hold this position for five seconds.

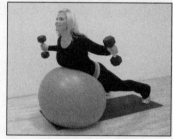

3. Lower the weights while draping your chest over the ball, and return to your starting position.

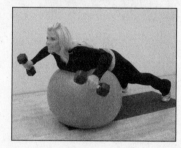

Do this for three sets of fifteen repetitions. Eventually increase the weight of the dumbbells.

One-Leg Lateral Shoulder Raises

What's happening: You will be working to develop pretty tank-top shoulders! Also, because you will have one leg raised, you will engage your abdominal muscles. (You need dumbbells for this exercise.)

1. Sit on the ball with your dumbbells resting at your side.

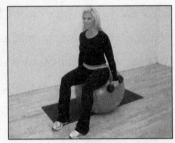

2. Lift one leg slightly off the floor.

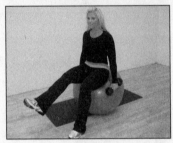

3. On the opposite side as your raised leg, pull the dumbbell up while keeping your elbow bent. Raise your arm until your elbow is level with your shoulder.

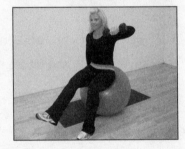

Lower and repeat ten times. Next, switch to the other side and lift the weight in the same way. Complete a total of two sets of ten repetitions. (Use two sets of dumbbells for this exercise. Begin with the lighter weight for the first set, and then increase the weight for the second set.)

Lying-Flat Ball Drops

What's happening: Both your upper and lower abs will be getting a great workout!

1. Lie on your back on the floor with your knees bent and your ankles and lower legs gripping the sides of the ball. Your arms will be flat on the floor, and your hands should be slightly underneath your bottom.

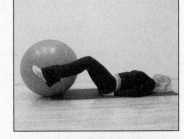

2. Grip the ball with your legs, concentrating on using your abdominal muscles to help lift the ball. Raise the ball until your legs are fully extended and the ball is suspended above your chin.

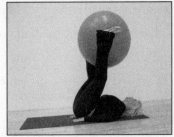

3. Lower the ball to the floor. However, do not allow your feet to touch the floor during each set.

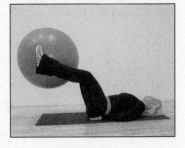

Complete a total of three sets, beginning with ten, twelve, and fifteen drops.

Exercises for Advanced Strength Training

Now you are advanced! This is an awesome place to be. You have done the work and put in some time, and you're ready to kick it up. By doing the five exercises that follow, you will take your conditioning and toning to a new level. Don't get discouraged if some of these are still difficult. Doing hard things is the key to getting superstrong!

Going for a Swim
What's happening: This move will feel like you are taking a swim minus the pool! It also will strengthen your back and shoulders.

1. Lie forward over the ball with your chest and torso resting on it. Your hips will be in the air, and your legs will be extended behind you.

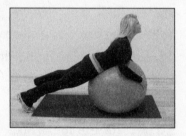

2. Extend your arms straight out in front and focus on creating a straight line with your body.

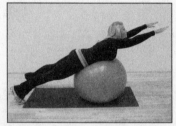

3. In a swimming and side-to-side motion, with your arms and fingertips extended, begin to twist your upper body. Only half of your chest will come off the ball at any time during this movement.

This exercise is more about the length of time you continue the motion than repetitions. Therefore, begin by completing twenty seconds. Work your way up to thirty seconds, then forty-five, then a full minute.

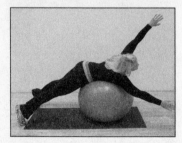

Push-up Leg Extensions

What's happening: This exercise may be the most difficult yet. Before you try it, practice holding the push-up position. The movement will strengthen every muscle group with an emphasis on the buttocks.

1. Lie over the ball with your body straight, keeping the area from your shins to your feet on the ball. Place your hands flat on the floor, a shoulder-width apart, and keep your arms straight. (This is the push-up position.)

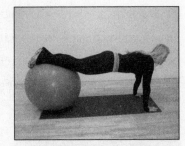

2. Lower your head slightly while maintaining a straight line with your body, and then lift one leg off the ball. (You will do this exercise with each leg being raised off the ball, but one at a time.)

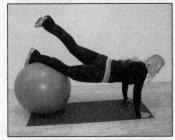

3. Bend your elbows and perform a push-up. Begin with five push-ups while each leg is lifted off the ball. Eventually work toward a total of three sets of ten repetitions with each leg.

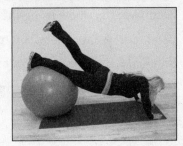

One-Arm, One-Leg Triceps Extensions

What's happening: This exercise will help tone the backs of your arms, the triceps. (You need dumbbells for this exercise.)

1. Lie with your back on the ball so that you are supporting your body weight from your feet to your waist. While holding a dumbbell in one hand, raise and extend the leg on the opposite side so it is pointing out straight in front of you.

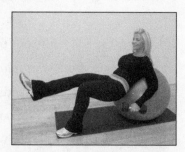

2. Raise the hand that is holding the weight until your arm is pointed nearly straight up in the air. You will need to focus on balancing your entire body on the ball.

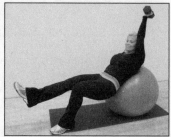

3. With the arm extended straight overhead, bend back the elbow using the triceps muscle to push the weight back into the starting position. Repeat for a total of ten repetitions on the first side. Switch sides and repeat.

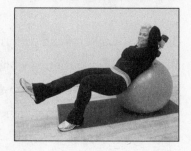

Do this for a total of three sets of ten repetitions on each arm. Increase the amount of weight with each set.

Frog Squats

What's happening: Primarily you will be toning and conditioning your buttocks, hamstrings, and quadriceps. You also will strengthen your ankle and knee joints. But be aware right off the bat that these squats will be hard. This exercise is advanced and should not be done if you have an injury or damage to your knees.

1. Stand and hold the ball at chest level with your feet in a very wide stance. They will be slightly more than a hip-width apart.

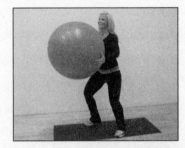

2. Hop like a frog with the ball in front of you. Be sure to use the power of your legs to get off the floor.

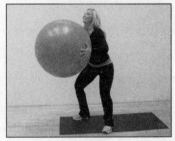

3. As you come down, drop your knees toward the floor and end up in a leaping position. Bring the ball down with you so it is only a few inches off the floor.

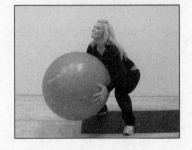

Do this for a total of two sets of ten repetitions. Your goal should be to get your feet off the floor higher and higher with practice.

Back-Bend Leg Kicks

What's happening: This final advanced move will challenge your spine, condition your upper and lower abs, and strengthen your upper body and lower body at the same time! Be patient. No matter how long it takes, you can get there. Once you are able to do this move, you will feel like you are building a very strong body.

1. Lie back on the ball so that it is beneath your waist, lower back, and buttocks. Raise your arms above your head and reach back to the floor. Do a back bend so that you are touching the floor with both hands and have both feet flat on the floor.

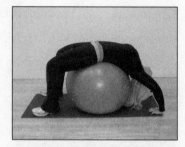

2. While balancing your body on the ball, lift your legs up as you maintain a slight bend in your knees.

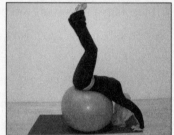

3. Straighten out one leg at a time while pulling in the opposite knee. Repeat with alternate leg.

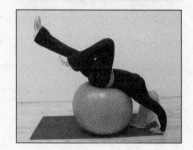

Complete this action for a total of fifteen seconds. Eventually complete three sets of fifteen, twenty, and thirty seconds total. Hurrah!

STRETCHING YOUR SUCCESS

In the past, when it came to stretching, I was guilty of complacency at times. But as I became a trainer and studied methods of stretching and the reasons behind it, I realized the error of my ways.

Think about this for a minute. Those of us who work out regularly are constantly contracting all our muscle groups. Muscles cover our bones and are composed of thousands of fibers and tendons. Without lengthening them and extending them prior to an exercise session, we risk injury.

Here's a vivid illustration. Grab a lime and squeeze it as tightly as you can. If some juice comes out, don't worry. It may help to make my point. Hold it supertight for a few minutes. Let go just a tiny bit and then repeat. Let go again just a little, and repeat. One more time.

Don't you want to put the lime down so you can extend your fingers? If you avoid stretching before you exercise, it's similar to holding that lime tightly for days on end. Honestly, you'd probably end up with arthritis.

This applies to all muscle groups and even the spine. Various cultures have been aware of this fact for many years. In the early 1900s, Joseph Pilates developed his own stretching methods. Pilates, as his technique came to be known, is used in the world of dance, gymnastics, and circus acrobatics. In fact, it has become somewhat of a household name as men and women who are looking to improve their health and physique practice it today.

The spine is responsible for many important functions in your body. The bones in your spine protect your spinal cord, the foundation of your central nervous system. Your spine also supports your upper body and enables you to stand up, bend, and twist. The backbone is the core of the body. Keeping this important part of your body flexible will help ensure the rest of your body is strong, including muscles and the entire nervous system.

Some of the benefits of stretching are that it offers more mobility, which improves all your exercise performance. Further, it improves your posture. Stretching also encourages optimum mental health by stimulating the nervous system and invigorating internal organs. Studies show that stretching can relieve menstrual pain and constipation.

Living well is about feeling incredible! The stretches I will show you are excellent to do before bedtime. They can help you fall asleep more quickly, because you will feel more relaxed. Sometimes it helps to do your stretching in a quiet place with soft music playing in the background. Once a week it could be a treat to make this happen. In fact, try inviting a few friends over to do some stretching together.

The following stretches are designed to include the entire body. Initially aim to hold each stretch for a minimum of fifteen seconds. Eventually, stretching in sequences of three sets is optimal. For example, try fifteen-, twenty-, and thirty-second increments for each one. You will find this plan to deliver the most improvements in flexibility. Remember, stretching should not be painful! When you are first doing these stretches, getting into the stretching position may feel uncomfortable for a few seconds. However, the stretch should begin to feel good as blood and energy are forced into your muscles.

Upper Body Stretches

Neck Stretch

Hang one arm by your side and then twist it so the palm is facing out, away from your body. With the other hand, grasp your head and pull it down toward that shoulder until your ear touches. Do this slowly and gently, and stop when you start to feel discomfort. Repeat with the other side.

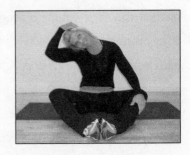

Shoulder Stretch

Place one arm across the front of your body. With the opposite hand, grasp your elbow. Now pull your arm across your body without twisting your torso. You should feel the tension in the front of your shoulder and possibly in the chest area. Switch arms and repeat.

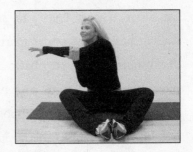

Triceps Stretch

Raise one hand above your head and then bend your elbow and place it behind your back. Place the other hand on the triceps muscle as pictured, and then begin to press the entire arm you are stretching while applying pressure with the hand on your back. Next, repeat on the opposite arm.

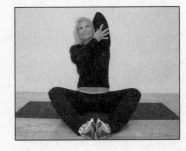

Spine Stretch

Stand with your feet hip-distance apart. Interlace your fingers and slowly bend forward at the waist while pressing your hands away from your chest. Do this until your back is parallel to the ground. As you hold the stretch, envision being able to balance a can of soda on your back. In other words, your 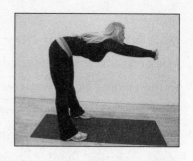 resting position for the stretch should produce a flat back, similar to a tabletop.

Chest Stretch

Stand and face a wall with your feet spread hip-distance apart. Place your hands on the wall at chest height, wider apart than shoulder distance. Next, step back and begin to press into the wall with your hands. Allow only your upper body to support your body weight. While holding this position, concentrate on contracting your chest muscles for the duration of the stretch.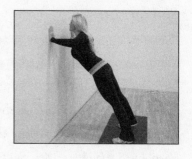

Hamstring Stretch

Lie on your back on the floor with your knees bent and your feet flat on the floor. Straighten one leg and lift it by placing both hands around the ankle and pulling up. Be sure to keep that leg straight as you stretch it. You should feel it pulling along the entire back of this leg. Switch legs and repeat the steps.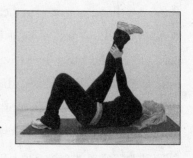

Quadriceps Stretch

Lie on your side. Using your free hand, reach behind you to pull up the leg on the same side by grasping the front of the foot. As you pull the foot upward and back toward your bottom, turn your knee at an angle. You should feel the stretch along the front of your leg and thigh. Alternate sides and legs and follow the same steps.

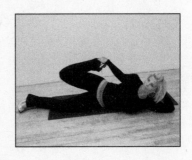

Calves Stretch

Kneel with one leg extended in front of you and the other leg behind you with your knee on the floor. Slowly lean forward while gently pulling your toes up and allowing the heel to press down. A comfortable stretch should be felt in the calf. Next perform this same movement on the opposite side.

Part 5

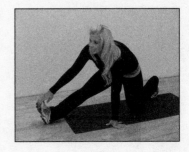

Living Well for the Rest of Your Life

16

Brownies, Birthdays, Cruises, Celebrations

How You Can Relax the Rules 20 Percent of the Time

I want to sweet-talk you. Literally. It's time to talk about things like brownies, birthday cake, and chocolate fountains. (If you have never seen a chocolate fountain, you are missing out.) Remember in the movie *Willy Wonka and the Chocolate Factory* how the river of chocolate ran through this little world? I'm pretty sure it was the inspiration for the popular chocolate fountain. Picture this confectionary contraption at the dessert table as it constantly flows with milky, creamy chocolate! Alongside it is an assortment of treats for dipping: strawberries, pretzels, pound cake, mini–Rice Krispies Treats, and more. It's really yummy and really addictive, so watch out!

But hold on a minute. As I'm typing these words, I need to stop and take a bite of something that is just as spectacular and right in front of me: a sensational salad! This salad has so many tasty treats in it that it's hard to keep track of them. They may not be as sweet as a brownie, but, honestly, they seem just as delightful.

My rainbow of nature's treasures has a bed of gorgeous mixed greens and several varieties of lettuce. The leafy greens lie on the bottom for my favorite, hand-selected valuables to rest on. An entire crunchy cucumber is sliced to perfection and sprawled across the top. Beautiful bright red cherry tomatoes blossom in this luxury salad as well. I couldn't enjoy this delicacy without broccoli, which resembles a bountiful bouquet. The garbanzo beans add terrific texture, and the onions pop in my mouth as I crunch. The light touch of balsamic dressing adds a richness that is tasty and tart. It offers unity to all the fabulous flavors.

I'm not pulling a bait-and-switch. When I talk about loving food, I'm referring to all foods. I consider the salad I'm eating to be a delicious treat, an amazing gift from God.

HOW DO YOU THINK ABOUT FOOD?

I didn't always think about all foods this way. In the years I fought obesity, my first loves were banana splits and chili cheese fries. Then I read an article that helped give me an entirely new perspective on food. As I worked to lose weight, I knew that changing the way I thought about things, food included, would mean the difference between regaining the weight I'd lost and keeping it off for good. Part of the fitness program I created was learning a new way to think about nutrition and my attachment to food.

This may come as a surprise to many, but it's not that difficult to derive great pleasure from eating healthy, energy-packed, nonglamorous food. You can gain a great deal of enjoyment from healthy flavors. I can't think of many meals I enjoy more than my creative, colorful lunchtime salad.

Now that I have maintained my target weight for many years, I have started to wonder, *Why can't I love all food like I love a salad?* When I was overweight, I was conflicted about food. I'd eat too much of it but rarely get the full pleasure of it, because I felt guilty about what I was eating. Even after I lost two hundred pounds, I still felt bound to this warped logic.

Have you ever watched a two-year-old eat an Oreo cookie? A toddler will nibble at the corners, break the cookie in half, slowly lick out the sweet center cream, and eventually eat each of the outer chocolate cookies, all the while obviously enjoying every bite. Now, contrast an adult's approach. Most people pop the cookie in their mouth and have the entire thing chewed and swallowed in the time it takes the two-year-old to figure out how to break it apart. Adults can gobble a half dozen in a matter of minutes. So rather than having the pleasure of one cookie, a grownup ends up feeling guilty about eating too many.

Motivating Emotions

Our eating habits tell us as much about ourselves as they do about the food we reach for when we're hungry. Even when we get control of our eating and start eating healthy, we still have an attachment to certain foods. Some form of emotional eating is always going to exist.

Think about this: even when you are disciplined about what and how much you eat while losing weight, emotions are still involved. As you make progress with your weight loss, your eating will be driven by the emotion that comes from wanting not to be overweight. It's a legitimate goal and certainly should motivate you to change your habits so you can change your life. But eventually we all need to approach food apart from our emotional connection to it.

Why can't we use food as a gift God has given us and learn how to love it with the emotion of controlled gratification? This brings me back to the deal of a lifetime. Have you noticed that everything we've talked about—cardio exercise, strength training, surrendering to God, and good nutrition—is connected to the deal of a lifetime, the deal that God offers us? God wants this for us even more than we want it for ourselves. He wants us to love food and live well. After all, if it weren't for God, we would have neither food nor life.

Loving Food and Living Well

What happens when we love food in the wrong way, and what changes when we love food in a way that helps us live well? Like many people, I love brownies. So what happens now when I want a brownie? I have one. But because I'm living well, I don't allow myself to have a brownie every day. When I do have one, I want to really love eating it. If I go overboard with brownies, I know that the pleasure will diminish. And with a brownie, it's worth it to get maximum enjoyment.

This is true with just about anything you love to eat. I love parties. I plan them, organize them, decorate for them, and enjoy them fully. And part of the celebration is eating special things. Birthday cake is yummy. When you're living well, you can have birthday cake. You also can partake in dipping strawberries in the chocolate fondue when you take that once-in-a-lifetime Caribbean cruise. Food is a gift to be enjoyed, but you need to have some ground rules, a set system.

At first it may seem a little awkward to do this, because we have become accustomed to popping too many things into our mouths simply because they look pretty and smell great. Before we realize it, we have chewed them, swallowed them, and maybe even grabbed for more. The irony is that in trying to enjoy it too much, we keep ourselves from enjoying it very much.

So how can we take more pleasure in the foods we eat?

I'll tell you. Here are ten things you might not be expecting, but they will revolutionize the way you eat, and they will deliver more enjoyment from eating than you thought possible. Some of them will take some practice, but they all will add up to more enjoyment as you learn to really love food.

1. Smile While You Swallow

This might not work with liver, so make sure you are eating something that can make you smile when you are swallowing it.

2. Feel Free to Spit It Out

If what you thought you wanted to eat looks good but tastes terrible, spit it out. If you hear your mother's voice telling you this is rude, just blame me. You can do this tastefully, by the way: raise your napkin to your mouth and deposit the food as you cover your mouth. If it's not worth eating, get rid of it.

3. Take the Time to Discover Great Food

It's worth the investment of time to become familiar with the colors and varieties of fresh fruits and vegetables. Purchase new, untried foods for your family to sample each week.

4. Close the Menu

If you're eating out and can't decide what to order within two minutes, close the menu and order a salad with grilled chicken. Most likely nothing seemed especially good, and you know in advance that the salad will taste great.

5. Believe the First Few Bites Are Where It's At

Remember, the idea is to get maximum enjoyment from food. So don't miss out on the first few bites, which are the most satisfying, no matter what you're eating. Don't be embarrassed to ask for a tiny bowl at the beginning to help you practice this. You can transfer a few bites of the treat into a small container, such as a bowl, to practice enjoying decadence in moderation. By taking a smaller portion, you will be more likely to savor the taste slowly.

6. Don't Let the Party Be on Your Plate

Some people have told me that they stopped going to parties because they had trouble walking away from the food being served. Their mistake was thinking that parties are about food. Not so. A party is a party because people you care about have gathered to share the enjoyment of a special occasion, not because fabulous food is being shared. Food should complement a gathering, not define it. I sometimes remind myself of this when I'm planning gatherings.

7. Food Can Go to Waste

You're not being righteous when you eat something simply because it's sitting there. I know if you could deliver it to a third-world nation, you would. But you can't, so it's better for the food to sit in the trash than to show up on your figure.

8. Know When Enough Is Enough

You are learning to get maximum pleasure from food, but that pleasure is containable and controllable. This means you will have the opportunity to enjoy food again tomorrow and the next day. Don't allow yourself to feel cheated or deprived. In other words, don't look at the piece of cheesecake as if you'll never see another one for the rest of your life. If you start to think this is the last piece of cheesecake on the planet, stop yourself and say, "Enough is enough." Say it out loud if you need to. As you have already heard from me, calories are the bottom line with any type of food we eat. If you have already had a day's worth of calories when you spot some cheesecake, exercise your freedom to postpone the cheesecake for another day. If you're limiting your calories to 2,000 per day, you exercised your free will earlier that day in choosing other foods. So try again tomorrow or next week.

9. Full Is Full

It dawned on me that I can feel just as full from a grilled chicken sandwich as I can from a Big Mac. So when I'm ravenous because I failed to space out my calories for the day or because I had an extra strenuous workout, I eat light and large. This means I usually have something that gives me a good quantity of food without a crazy amount of calories. I just need to be full, and I can do that without overdosing on wasteful calories. Chicken, a salad, and some sweet potato will usually do the trick.

10. Close Your Eyes

Shut your eyes for ten seconds when you are eating something you really want, every time if possible. Remind yourself that food is a gift. Allow yourself to be aware of the flavors in it. Say a short prayer and be thankful for the opportunity to enjoy such pleasure.

As you can see, when you practice these ten ways to get maximum enjoyment from food, you will have to do things differently than you have in the past. But that's a big part of living well. If you were dissatisfied with your life before, and you desire a new way of living, it makes sense that you have to start doing things differently. The result is a different life—the life you have been hoping for all along.

We started this book by saying that we can indeed love food and live well. We have covered good nutrition, a practical weight-loss plan, cardio fitness, and strength training. We have addressed our spirit as well, discussing the necessity of seeking God's help, being grateful for His care for us, and surrendering our lives to His strength, love, and power. That is how we all can live well. And we can get more enjoyment from food than ever before while still eating clean and either losing weight or maintaining the healthy weight we have achieved.

WHAT TO DO WHEN YOU BLOW IT

By now you have experienced some big breakthroughs with diet, nutrition, and exercise. You might have already noticed a smaller number when you step on the scales. I applaud your progress. I hope you are growing in confidence that you can fully accept and benefit from God's deal of a lifetime.

It would be wonderful to believe that once you read this book, you will no longer struggle with the dark clouds of depression and frustration over your self-esteem, body image, and weight. I won't try to sell you that deal, because we are both committed to telling the truth. Instead, I can only offer what God has shown me and told me to share with you. It's a matter of hope, promise, truth, and peace. Over time you will achieve your goals, but it won't always be steady, uninterrupted progress. Life is unpredictable, and other things will get in the way from time to time. At some point you will blow it. Since you're human, you'll make mistakes. You will be disappointed. Know these things are coming, but don't let yourself be deceived, defeated, or defined by them. Circumstances will work against you, but there is always hope. You as a person are not a mistake or a disappointment. You can overcome the obstacles you face and the occasional failure to stick to your commitment.

A few years ago I was driving along the Sawgrass Expressway in South Florida. I was headed home after doing some holiday shopping, and I found myself anxious to get off the highway and to rest my weary feet. As I was zipping along, nearing my exit, I heard a loud noise. Immediately I began to veer off the road. With all my strength I tried to regain control of my car. I was trying to keep it on a straight line, but the car was swerving toward the shoulder. It was intense—definitely one of those "had to be there" moments.

I was shaking inside and screaming out loud, "Dear God! Dear God!" as I managed to steer my car off the road. Sure, it was superscary. But I survived it. I was alive and well, thank God.

I sat in the car for a few minutes with my head down and cried with sheer thankfulness. This situation could have been the end for me, but it wasn't. The next thing I did was get out of the car to figure out what had gone wrong. It took less than a minute to realize the problem. One of my tires had blown.

I'm pretty clueless about mechanical things. I know you need a jack and a spare, but that's the extent of my knowledge. So I made a phone call to the experts. It didn't take long for AAA to get there. The man who showed up told me that he fixes cars all day long. I was very grateful I had someone to call.

What does my broken-down car have to do with your learning to love food and live well every day of your life? Everything, really! You see, when my tire blew and I finally pulled the car off the road, I didn't have the option to just quit driving. Imagine if I had called my husband and said, "Babe, the car broke down. I blew a tire. I think we should just scrap this vehicle." Yet when we mess up in life, especially in the care of our bodies, we are tempted to scrap our health instead of assessing the problem and fixing it.

That night, with a flat tire and little idea of how to put on the spare, I did the smartest thing I knew to do: I called for help. You need to do the same thing every time you blow it. I have blown it myself. I've had a few too many cookies at Christmas. I've also kept eating after the food has lost its taste. I have cut short a few workouts because I just didn't feel like exercising that day. But the difference is that I refuse to let my human flaws and shortcomings cause me to fail. I will not sacrifice the freedom I have.

God has given us the freedom to make choices, decisions, and commitments. That freedom is one of His greatest gifts to us. So whenever you blow it, make the decision to get back up and get with the program. It's your choice, so use your freedom to your best advantage.

There was a major headline in the news a few years ago. Every time I logged on to the Internet it was there: Oprah Winfrey admitted she had gained forty pounds. Shocking as this news was (I know hardly anyone else had noticed Oprah's weight gain), I was moved by her candor. She doesn't owe anyone an explanation. I have read that her television program's ratings will sometimes go up when she gains weight. Apparently this struggle humanizes her.

I have a theory about Oprah's honesty in talking about her struggles with gaining weight. Because she is an advocate for living well, I think she feels a sense of responsibility to own up to her shortcomings. Being honest and telling the truth—to ourselves and to others—is part of what is required in living well.

I may scream if I hear one more person say about Oprah's admission, "Well, if I had all her money, I'd…" My response is, "You'd what? Pay someone to hop on the elliptical for you? Have someone lock you in a room at night so you couldn't grab a late-night snack?" Come on, money doesn't fix any area of personal weakness. If anything, it encourages it. People who have plenty of money will spend it as they keep looking for the joy they are desperate to find.

Having money or not having it has nothing to do with living well. Nor does it affect your ability to choose to get back up after failing, after falling down, after messing up. I know about failing and wanting to give up. And I know about God's strength in helping me choose to try again. Without the hope that God gives me, I would have given up for good a long time ago.

I'm thankful for the desperation I felt that night ten years ago when I surrendered to God. I was driving home from a meeting, and, honestly, I had run out of reasons to live. Because I had blown it so many times, I had nothing left but to ask The Expert.

I was so overweight that if I didn't change my life, I was headed for an early death. I was so miserable that even though I was alive physically, my soul was in turmoil. Proverbs 16:25 reminds us about the consequences of going down a path on our own. "There is a way that seems right to a man, but in the end it leads to death" (NIV). This is why, when you blow it in any area of life, you won't be able to fix it on your own. You need help from outside.

The day I blew a tire driving on the Sawgrass Expressway, if I hadn't called for help, I'd still be sitting there on the side of the road, stranded and annoyed. None of us can handle setbacks and pain alone. My heart broke for Oprah when I read about her coming out about her weight gain. I wanted to hang out with her, just to hug her and say, "I get it, my friend." Oprah and I don't need to agree on everything in life to understand each other, because pain is universal.

RELIEF FROM THE PAIN OF FAILURE

If you had suffered from a disease, perhaps some rare form of cancer, and you knew you had found a cure, you'd want to scream it from the rooftops. Right? On most days this is how I feel when I wake up. I can barely contain my joy and excitement for the miracle I know is waiting for so many.

When you blow it—and you will—I want you to remember the following words:

> Are you tired? Worn out? Burned out on religion? Come to me. Get away with me and you'll recover your life. I'll show you how to take a real rest. Walk with me and work with me—watch how I do it. Learn the unforced rhythms of grace. I won't lay anything heavy or ill-fitting on you. Keep company with me and you'll learn to live freely and lightly. (Matthew 11:28–30, MSG)

Doesn't that sound like the best answer for anytime you mess up? You can ditch religious thinking that may tell you you're not good enough, and you can hand over all your pain and burden to the only One who has the power to grant you the grace to survive the struggle. The One who wants to help you is the God of the universe.

Whenever I blow it with food, there is one quick way I recover. I give it up! Seriously, I stop eating for a day. You can try this too. (It won't damage your metabolism in just twenty-four hours.) Take a break from food by making it a time of fasting. This will be only a temporary plug, but it will get you back on track again. As you acknowledge your mistake and incorporate prayer and positive thinking into a day of fasting, you will gain newfound strength, and you'll be able to fly down the road to living well.

When I began writing this chapter, I was enjoying a delicious salad. I'm now preparing to take a stroll in Manhattan, where I came on a business trip. And while I'm out, I think I'll search for something sweet. I promise you I won't settle on something just because it looks good. I'll make sure it's well worth the calories, and if not, it's in the trash! Deal?

Epilogue

Live Well in the Sweet Land of Liberty

ost days I don't go looking for adventure, but some-how one finds me. My life is a great adventure, and today is no exception." If these words sound familiar, it may be because I wrote them in the introduction to this book quite some time ago. And from where I sit today, they are ever so true!

With my hectic schedule and family life, writing requires my getting away for a few days. While some writers lock themselves away for months, I can't roll that way. Every day I need to see people, meet people, smile at people, and see them smile back. I love people.

So instead of months spent in a cabin, I steal four or five days at a time and operate on little sleep and loads of green tea. I'm a bit sad when I leave my husband and the kids, but the cool thing is that they understand. It's a matter of my using a gift from God and helping the hopeless with the words

He gives me to write. With my family's encouragement, I have a bounty of strength to press on and stay the course.

As I was completing work on this book, I knew beyond a shadow of a doubt that I needed to get back to New York to finish my writing. If you remember the beginning, when I introduced the deal of a lifetime, I was writing on my laptop while sitting on a bench a block away from Wall Street. It seemed amazingly appropriate to be writing about loving food and living well from the view I had that day. Wall Street symbolizes gigantic deals, and in this book we've talked about the deals we are offered. In the past we have bought into the world's deal, but now we know about the deal of a lifetime, which is much, much bigger than anything being traded on Wall Street.

Back then, I ended up on Wall Street because of a canceled flight and some fancy online hotel bidding. When I felt God nudge me to finish my writing back in New York, I had time to plan ahead and pick my spot. I wanted a private, quiet place, so I rented an apartment from a nice Russian woman in the city. (Yes, there is a Web site where you can find apartments for short-term rental. It can save lots of money and deliver much more space than a hotel room.)

When I arrived, the weather was cold, windy, and rainy. My umbrella got caught in a gust of wind that turned it into a pretzel as I was climbing out of a cab. I walked into the lobby of the building and looked around. Every couch in the lobby, and I'm talking about fifteen of them, was upholstered in a beautiful velvet butterfly fabric. I had never seen anything like it. Butterflies on couches? Everywhere I look?

You won't believe how excited I was. I had just written a song about God and the transformation of my life. The song is called "You Give Me Butter-flies." As I stood in the lobby of my temporary New York home, I said, "Thank You, Lord. You brought me here!"

I headed up to the apartment to meet the woman from whom I was renting. She greeted me with a warm smile, and while I checked out the place, she slipped in a surprise. "I'm sorry. There is no longer Internet or television available here. The building went digital a few days ago, and I haven't signed up for the service yet."

Oh, come on, I thought. *You must be joking.* I was freezing, tired, and more than ready to relax and get down to writing. So I hated the idea of hunting for another place to stay, but I had to have an Internet connection. I ended up at a hotel just a few blocks from Wall Street, in lower Manhattan. I paid no attention to the location when I chose it. I just had to find a place. I entered the lobby and felt nothing. There were no butterflies on the couches. Instead it was crowded and noisy, with lots of construction going on.

Crowded. Noisy construction. This was a far cry from a quiet apartment in a building with butterfly upholstery on the lobby couches. Why had I felt so much peace at the wrong place, only to have God bring me somewhere else?

Do you trust Me, daughter? I felt God asking.

Yes, Lord, but I'm annoyed.

I know. You are easily annoyed.

I checked in, received my room key card, and got on the elevator for the sixth floor. As soon as I opened the door, I felt relieved. I could finally set down my luggage after many hours of traveling. Also I was worn-out from the added accommodations drama.

I walked through the door and realized this was a suite. Cool. It had plenty of space, especially for a New York hotel room. As I headed into the bedroom, I saw two big windows. Opening the curtain, I hoped for a view. A pipe dream really.

I couldn't believe it. Instead of an alley or an air shaft, on one side I saw the Hudson River and Battery Park. And out the other window there she was, standing tall, seeming to say to me, "I'm so glad you're finally here." The Statue of Liberty.

Oh, Lord, why do You love me so much? I don't deserve all this. I had been annoyed. I even questioned You. I tried to figure out how I got it wrong even with all my planning.

His response: *Even with your trying to do all the right things and be more in control, you didn't truly have control. Because you let Me guide you, I brought you to the harbor. This harbor is a symbol of hope. This statue is a symbol of security and liberty. Tell them…tell them what only I can give.*

My dear friends, liberty is costly. And surrender is freedom. If you are ready to abandon all of your funk and failures, forgiveness is waiting. Freedom can be yours. Immigrants sought refuge in the waters of this harbor for hundreds of years. They made the choice to seek freedom and ended up in this foreign land full of hope. They desired freedom, so they pressed on through the fear of the unknown, all for the dream of finally becoming free.

A few months earlier, while hanging out with my kids on the beach in Florida, I met an elderly woman who told me she had been in a concentration camp. As I was writing this book, the memory of our conversation slipped my mind. That is, until this morning, the time I set aside to write this epilogue.

I'll never forget her asking me what I did for work, and I told her that in addition to being a mommy, I basically write about food. She responded, "I know what it is to be so desperate for something to eat, you'd do anything." I felt humbled. Here I am, telling her my life's work is to try to teach people to stop eating. And this survivor of the Holocaust had experienced the fear of losing her life because of not having any food.

She told me she tries to eat enough to fill her belly but not so much to make her stop appreciating food. This lovely Jewish woman represents the predicament we all face. How can we find the balance between fulfilling our needs and desires and not letting our desires control our needs? I know from my own past that this is the spot where we ultimately lose the dream of fulfilling both.

The answer to every dilemma will always be your acceptance of the deal of a lifetime. Go ahead, right now. Grab hold of the hand of God. No matter how many times you have let go in the past, tightly hold on to it today. Feel His grip. He wants you to know you don't ever need to let go again. With Him, the liberty to love food is yours. With Him, the liberty to live well will be the by-product of your choice to be free. So enter God's harbor and find refuge in the freedom He gives you. Forget for a moment what you are leaving behind and look at what is waiting.

As I gazed out my hotel window at our country's most famous statue and noticed all the activity on the street below, all I could think about was you. I knew the people who would read this book would come with questions and struggles and needs. I knew that, like me, you would come with hurts and past failures and a deep need for hope.

Won't you come along with me now? It's time for you to begin your own great adventure. And believe me, the view is worth it.

Dining Out Without Caving In

Restaurants these days are serving out-of-control portions! But eating out is something we all enjoy on occasion, so it's time to take charge. Use this new guide as a helpful tool when you find yourself overwhelmed with an endless menu in front of you and baskets of bread everywhere.

1. You Are in Control

Always remember the most important rule: You are always in control. You are under no obligation to eat something just because a server places it in front of you. The people in your life should not feel validated based on your eating habits and food selections when you are together! (And never forget that you are the only one who will wear the extra calories!)

2. WRAP IT UP

When you order, always ask for a separate plate. Then, as soon as the waiter brings your food, place half the portion on the extra plate and ask the server to wrap it up. Take it home and eat it the following day for lunch or dinner.

3. PAY ATTENTION TO PREPARATION

As you study a menu, pay close attention to how the food is going to be prepared. Stay clear of dishes that are described with words such as *buttered, battered, fried, glazed,* and *creamed.* Instead, look for words such as *baked* and *steamed.* Also, don't hesitate to specify how you want a certain dish to be cooked. You have the power to make sure your food is prepared in a healthier manner.

4. SALAD SIMPLY SATISFIES

When considering menu options, this is more helpful than any other trick. Never underestimate the power of salad. It fills you up, not out. That is mostly because of the high water content, but it's also because you end up chewing for a long time without taking in an insane amount of calories. After you've eaten a healthy salad you feel full—as if you've had a large meal. And if you're going to eat a full meal, have a salad before the main course. (Dressing should be light and on the side.) Best of all, you'll be less hungry when the entrée arrives.

5. SHARE

Senior citizens are brilliant when it comes to this one. They don't care if sharing one order with a friend might make them look cheap. It never hurts to share, even if you're *not* a senior. And it can do you a lot of good. So try this with a friend when you go out to dinner. Discuss what you both enjoy eating, order one of that item, and split it. If you're worried the server will receive an insufficient tip, add a few extra dollars. Not only will you save a few bucks, you'll save yourself a few hundred calories that you don't really need to feel satisfied.

6. The First Few Bites Are Magic

If there's one thing I've learned about having dessert after a meal, it's this: The first few bites are really the best. So if you're out for a celebration meal and dessert is in order, limit yourself to three bites and really savor them. This way you have the taste without the guilt! And remember rule No. 1: You are always in control.

NOTES

Chapter 3: The Barbie Myth Is the World's Deal

1. Ruth Handler, *Dream Doll: The Ruth Handler Story* (Stamford, CT: Longmeadow Press, 1994).

2. The Great Idea Finder, www.ideafinder.com/history/inventions/barbiedoll.

3. Data taken from a study conducted at the University of Missouri–Columbia, cited in "Women of All Sizes Feel Badly About Their Bodies After Seeing Models," *Science Daily,* March 27, 2007, www.sciencedaily.com/releases/2007/03/070326152704.htm.

4. Liz Dittrich, "About-Face Facts on Body Image," About-Face, www.about-face.org/r/facts/bi.shtml.

5. Lisa Berzins, "Dying to Be Thin: The Prevention of Eating Disorders and the Role of Federal Policy" (November 1997). The data was cited in a congressional briefing cosponsored by the American Psychological Association.

6. Susan Paxton et al., "Body Image Satisfaction, Dieting Beliefs, and Weight Loss Behaviors in Adolescent Girls and Boys," *Journal of Youth and Adolescence* 20 (1991): 361–79.

7. "Fast Facts: Media's Effect on Body Image," Teen Health and the Media, http://depts.washington.edu/thmedia/view.cgi?section=bodyimage&page=fastfacts.

Chapter 4: God Offers You the Deal of a Lifetime

1. Terry Britten and Graham Lyle, "What's Love Got to Do with It?" Capitol Records, 1984.

Chapter 6: Define Your Expectations Now!

1. Chantel Hobbs, *Never Say Diet: Make Five Decisions and Break the Fat Habit for Good* (Colorado Springs: WaterBrook, 2007), 76–81.
2. Helen McCormack, "The shape of things to wear: scientists identify how women's figures have changed in 50 years," *Independent* (London), November 21, 2005, www.independent.co.uk/news/uk/this-britain/the-shape-of-things-to-wear-scientists-identify-how-womens-figures-have-changed-in-50-years-516259.html.

Chapter 7: It's Time to Get a Clue About Calories

1. Roberta R. Friedman, "Scientific Studies Related to Menu Labeling," Yale University Rudd Center for Food Policy and Obesity, Menu Labeling: Opportunities for Public Policy, www.cspinet.org/new/pdf/yale_rudd_ctr_menu_labeling_grouped_studies.pdf.
2. Cited at James Beckerman, "Can't Read Food Labels? You're Not Alone," The Heart Beat, October 4, 2006, http://blogs.webmd.com/heart-disease/2006_10/cant-read-food-lables-youre-not-alone.html.
3. This information is included in NCHS Health E-Stat, "Prevalence of Overweight and Obesity Among Adults: United States, 2003–2004," National Center for Health Statistics, www.cdc.gov/nchs/data/hestat/overweight/overweight_adult_03.htm.
4. "The Golden Boy," *60 Minutes,* CBS, December 2, 2008, www.cbsnews.com/video/watch/?id=4639050n.

Chapter 8: Carbs: The First Temptation—Go Figure!

1. Answer key for the carb test in chapter 8 (S indicates a simple carbohydrate; C indicates a complex carbohydrate): orange (S), croissant (S), oatmeal (C), chewing gum (S), grape soda (S), cantaloupe (S), bagel (C), tortilla (C), doughnut (S), Cheerios (C), pretzels (S), strawberries (S), pasta (C), fudge (S), ice cream (S), honey (S), dark chocolate (S), saltines (S).

Chapter 9: Want Power? Eat Protein

1. "Mitigation Assessment Team Report: Hurricane Andrew in Florida," December 21, 1992, FEMA Resource Record Details, www.fema .gov/library/viewRecord.do?id=2765.
2. Elisa Zied, *So What Can I Eat? How to Make Sense of the New Dietary Guidelines for Americans and Make Them Your Own* (Hoboken, NJ: Wiley, 2006), 135.
3. Thomas L. Halton and Frank B. Hu, "The Effects of High Protein Diets on Thermogenesis, Satiety and Weight Loss: A Critical Review," *Journal of the American College of Nutrition* 23, no. 5 (2004): 373–85.

Chapter 10: Fat *Is Not a Four-Letter Word*

1. For more on this, see "Eat Well: Omega-3 and Omega-6 Fatty Acids: Getting the Balance You Need," Your Pathway to Wellness, Program of Northwestern Health Sciences University, www.nwhealth.edu/ healthyu/eatWell/omegas.html.
2. Artemis Simopoulos, "The Omega Plan," *Collins Living,* February 3, 1999, 67.

Chapter 11: How to Make Meals Meaningful

1. "Weight Loss and Breakfast: Breakfast Benefits Health and Can Aid in Weight Loss," Harvard Health Publications, Harvard Medical School, www.health.harvard.edu/press_releases/weight_loss_healthy_breakfast.htm.

Chapter 12: Today, Get Your New Life Moving

1. "Study: Most Americans Don't Exercise Regularly," CNN .com/Health, April 7, 2002, http://archives.cnn.com/2002/HEALTH/04/07/americans.exercise/index.html.

Chapter 14: How to "Bring It" with Interval Training

1. You might be more familiar with the standard formula for figuring heart-rate exercise goals that are often posted in fitness centers. It begins with subtracting your age from 220. The difference represents your maximum heart rate. Next, you use that number as you multiply certain percentages to arrive at different levels of exercise intensity. The problem with this formula is that it doesn't take into account your heart and your typical resting heart rate. Instead, it looks only at your age.